Renal Tubular Acidosis in Children

Ricardo Muñoz
Editor

Renal Tubular Acidosis in Children

New Insights in Diagnosis and Treatment

Springer

Editor
Ricardo Muñoz
Mexico City, Mexico

ISBN 978-3-030-91939-9   ISBN 978-3-030-91940-5 (eBook)
https://doi.org/10.1007/978-3-030-91940-5

This Springer imprint is published by the registered company Springer Nature Switzerland AG
The registered company address is: Gewerbestrasse 11, 6330 Cham, Switzerland

Completing this book was not possible without the participant authors, who enhanced the quality of the chapters with their outstanding knowledge in the field.

We dedicate this work to our spouses and children, who encouraged us enthusiastically, to continue our work diligently. We appreciate their patience and understanding when we, instead of spending our free time with them, used it to carry out this publication. We hope this book may be a reward to them.

My gratitude in a very special way to my wife Marisela for her support in every matter concerning my work.

I wish to thank my grandsons Ricardo and Guillermo, as well as my daughter Marisela for helping me with the technical support I needed to put this work altogether.

Also, we may use this space to the memory of our colleague Dr. Mario Matos-Martínez, co-author of the last chapter of the book. He passed away during the pandemic, which devastated so many people and colleagues around the world. Rest in peace.

Ricardo Muñoz, MD

Foreword

The purpose of this work is to spread recently acquired knowledge on renal physiology, which is applied to the clinical situation of a disease known as renal tubular acidosis (RTA). In this publication, we focus our attention on systemic and renal physiology related to renal tubular acidosis (RTA) in children. The clinical presentation, epidemiology, etiology, diagnosis, complications, and treatment bear different implications in children compared to those in the adult population. Besides, attention has been paid to many differences between adult and childhood physiologic mechanisms of handling systemic and renal acid-base metabolism, as well as fluid and electrolyte disturbances that are closely related to RTA.

Epidemiologically, RTA in the pediatric age group is a very rare disease. The incidence has been calculated to be as low as $1{:}10^6$ in the general population. RTA (despite being a very rare renal disease) has contributed like no other renal alteration to the knowledge of acid-base balance in Medicine, most likely due to the interest that has been aroused in the scenario of scientific research.

Great advances in the fields of genetics and molecular biology have established important modifications in our basic knowledge of systemic acid-base metabolism, as well as on the renal handling of hydrogen ions and bicarbonate, determined, in turn, by the action of protein transmembrane transporters located at the membranes of the renal tubular cells.

RTA is an entity of miscellaneous etiology, with physiologic situations not too easy to understand, which reflects the complexity of acid-base metabolism involved in the pathology of RTA.

The complications that result in the different types of RTA further complicate the situation, since they involve other organs, besides the kidneys. Endocrine, metabolic, and fluids and electrolytes alterations are quite common in children with RTA. Alterations in sodium, chloride, potassium, calcium, and phosphates metabolism, among others, are evident, especially those which affect the production and secretion of parathyroid hormone, vitamin D, calcium sensor-receptor, renin-angiotensin-aldosterone-endothelin system, thyroid hormones, and antidiuretic hormone.

These alterations represent a deleterious impact, especially on sexual maturation, as well as in growth and development, so important in the pediatric age group.

Furthermore, the alterations described in some types of RTA have led to the development of significant sequelae, such as kidney stone formation and nephrocalcinosis, which in turn, facilitate the appearance of repeated urinary tract infections and progression into chronic kidney interstitial damage and end-stage renal failure.

We hope the scientific compilation provided herein may help as an aid in the understanding of the physiology of RTA in children and contribute to the diagnosis, management, and treatment of this entity.

Mexico City, Mexico Ricardo Muñoz

Preface

One of the main motivations for this publication was a sudden increase in children falsely diagnosed as having RTA. This problem began and spread more than a decade ago in some Latin American countries. A careful review of several cases with a recent diagnosis of RTA revealed that the overall had an incorrect diagnosis since the clinical and laboratory data found in the clinical records did not support the evidence of the diagnosis of RTA.

The inappropriate diagnosis of RTA in children happens in hospital settings and private practice. Dozens of these children were contacted and studied again by expert pediatric nephrologists under the appropriate and supervised laboratory diagnostic technology, concluding there was an overdiagnosis of RTA.

Even though some publications were made on this matter in the medical literature, the problem of overdiagnosis of RTA has been increasing to this day.

Therefore, this work intends to reach general practitioners, gastroenterologists, endocrinologists, healthcare personnel, and, especially, pediatricians and growth and development services that are the first contact with children with the main feature of RTA, which is failure to thrive. Therefore, they may be able to find in this publication the scientific information to make up the correct diagnosis and, if necessary, refer patients to the pediatric nephrologist to achieve this purpose. Unfortunately, some pediatric nephrologists continue to support the mistaken diagnosis of RTA which, in turn, may explain the expansion of this false "epidemic" of renal tubular acidosis in children.

Besides, it is important to alert the general population on this matter, hoping to avoid the risk of making repeatedly an incorrect diagnosis of RTA and the undesirable effects of prolonged treatment, as well as the emotional and economic burden of a misdiagnosis. All this is coupled with the ethical implications and possible consequences of legal liability.

The initial chapters include a review of the basic principles of systemic metabolism of hydrogen and carbon dioxide and sodium bicarbonate in states of health and disease, focusing the attention on the pediatric population. These chapters include a review of the renal physiology related to the regulation of acid-base metabolism. The following chapters describe the different types of RTA, the etiology, pathophysiology, diagnosis, and, treatment, paying special attention to the molecular basis of protein transmembrane transporters working at hydrogen excretion and bicarbonate tubular reabsorption in different tubular cells of the nephron.

Mexico City, Mexico

Ricardo Muñoz

Contents

Contributors

Patricia Tejera Carreño, MD Pediatric Emergency Service, University Hospital, Hospital Universitario Insular Materno Infantil, Las Palmas de Gran Canaria, Canary Islands, Spain

María Castañeda-Bueno, MD Departamento de Nefrología y Metabolismo Mineral, Instituto Nacional de Ciencias Médicas y Nutrición Salvador Zubirán, Mexico City, México

Laura Escobar-Pérez, PhD Department of Physiology, Faculty of Medicine, National Autonomous University of Mexico, Mexico City, Mexico

National Autonomous University of Mexico, Mexico City, Mexico

National System of Investigators, Mexico City, Mexico

Gerardo Gamba, MD Departamento de Nefrología y Metabolismo Mineral, Instituto Nacional de Ciencias Médicas y Nutrición Salvador Zubirán, Mexico City, México

Víctor M. García Nieto, MD Pediatric Nephrology Section of the University Hospital Nuestra Señora de Candelaria, Santa Cruz de Tenerife, Canary Islands, Spain

Omar Guadarrama, MD Research and Diagnosis of Nephrology and, Bone Mineral Metabolism, Hospital Infantil de México Federico Gómez, Mexico City, Mexico

Norma Elizabeth Guerra Hernández, MD Department of Pediatric Nephrology, General "Dr. Gaudencio González Garza," National Medical Center La Raza, Mexican Institute of Social Security, Mexico City, Mexico

Advanced Studies Iztacalaca Faculty, National Autonomous University of Mexico, Mexico City, Mexico

Jesús Lagunas-Muñoz, MD Department of Pediatric Nephrology, National Medical Center La Raza, Mexican Institute of Social Security, Mexico City, Mexico

High Specialty Medical Unit, General Hospital "Dr. Gaudencio González Garza." National Medical Center La Raza, Mexican Institute of Social Security, Mexico City, Mexico

Mario Matos-Martínez, MD Pediatric Nephrology Service, Medical Unit of High Specialty National Medical Center La Raza, Mexican Institute of Social Security, Mexico City, Mexico

Faculty of Medicine, National Autonomous University of Mexico, Mexico City, Mexico

Mara Medeiros, MD Research and Diagnosis of Nephrology and, Bone Mineral Metabolism, Hospital Infantil de México Federico Gómez, Mexico City, Mexico

Faculty of Medicine, National Autonomous University of Mexico, Mexico City, Mexico

National System of Investigators, Level III, Mexico City, Mexico

Teresa Moraleda Mesa, MD Canary Islands, Spain

Ricardo Muñoz, MD Retired from: Department of Pediatric Nephrology, Hemodialysis Unit, The Children's Hospital at Albany Medical Center, Albany, NY, USA

Retired from: Pediatric Nephrology Department, Hospital Infantil de México Federico Gómez, Mexico City, Mexico

Retired from: Research Division, Hospital Infantil de Mexico Federico Gomez, Mexico City, Mexico

Retired from: National System of Investigators, Level I, Mexico City, Mexico

Retired from: North American Pediatric Renal Transplantation Collaborative Study (NAPRTCS) Study, Woburn, MA, USA

Adrián Rafael Murillo-de-Ozores, MD Departamento de Nefrología y Metabolismo Mineral, Instituto Nacional de Ciencias Médicas y Nutrición Salvador Zubirán, Mexico City, México

Rosa Vargas-Poussou, MD, PhD Département de Génetique, Hôpital Européen Georges Pompidou, Paris, France

María Isabel Luis Yanes, MD Section of Pediatric Nephrology, University Hospital of Nuestra Señora de Candelaria, Santa Cruz de Tenerife, Canary Islands, Spain

Javier Zamora-García, MD Division of Pediatrics, Hospital Central Norte, Servicios Medicos de Petroleos Mexicanos, Mexico City, Mexico

Faculty of Medicine, National Autonomous University of Mexico, Mexico City, Mexico

Margarita Monge Zamorano, MD Pediatric Nephrology Section of the University Hospital Nuestra Señora de Candelaria, Santa Cruz de Tenerife, Canary Islands, Spain

Abbreviations

(NH_3)	Ammonia
(NH_4^+)	Ammonium
(nm/l)	Nano-moles per Liter
(OH^-)	Hydroxyl Ions
[H^+]	Hydrogen Ion (Proton) Concentration
[HCO_3^-]	Bicarbonate Concentration
11-β-HSD2	11-β-Hydroxysteroid Dehydrogenase Type II
ACTH	Adrenocorticotropin Hormone
ADH	Antidiuretic Hormone
AII RB	Angiotensin II type I Receptor Blockers
AQP	Aquaporin
ASDN	Aldosterone-Sensitive Distal Nephron
BK	Maxi-K Channels
CA II/IV	Carbonic Anhydrase 2 and 4
CaSR	Calcium Sensor-Receptor
CCT	Cortical Collecting Duct
CNT	Connecting Tubule
DOC	Deoxycorticosterone
DRTA	Distal Renal Tubular Acidosis
ECF	Extracellular Fluid
ENaC	Epithelial Sodium Channels
FENa	Fractional Na^+ Excretion of Sodium
GH	Growth Hormone
GTTK	Renal Trans-tubular Potassium Gradient
H^+ATPase (V-H^+ATPase)	Hydrogen Pump; Hydrogen Adenosine-Triphosphatase (Vacuolar Hydrogen Pump)
H^+K^+ATPase	Hydrogen Ion/Potassium Exchanger
H_2CO_3	Carbonic Acid
HCN1-HCN4	Hyperpolarization-Activated Cation Channels and Cyclic Nucleotides (Pacemaker Channels)
HCO_3^-	Bicarbonate

HFABP	Cardiac Fatty Acid-Binding Protein
ICF	Intracellular Fluid
IF	Intercellular Fluid
IGF-1	Insulin-Like Growth Factor
K^+/Cl^-	Potassium/Chloride Exchanger (Anti-transporter)
kAE1	Anionic Anti-transporter (HCO_3^-/Cl^-)
KIM-1	Kidney Damage Molecule-1
L-FABP	Protein Fatty Acid Binding
mmHg	Millimeters of Mercury
MR	Mineralocorticoid Receptor
Na^+/K^+ATPase	Basolateral Sodium/Potassium Pump; Sodium-Potassium Adenosine-Triphosphatase)
$Na^+K^+2Cl^-$	Sodium/Potassium/Chloride Cotransporter
NBCe1-NBC3	Basolateral Membrane Sodium/Bicarbonate Exchanger (Anti-transporter)
NCC	Thiazide-Sensitive Sodium-Chloride Cotransporter
$NH_4^+Cl^-$	Ammonium Chloride
NHE3	Luminal Na^+H^+ Exchanger (Anti-transporter)
NKCC2 (NKCC1)	Cotransporter Na^+ K^+ $2Cl^-$
NSAID	Nonsteroidal Anti-inflammatory Drugs
OMCD	Outer Medullary Collecting Duct
pCO_2	Carbon Dioxide Partial Pressure
PGE_2	Prostaglandins
pH	Negative Logarithm of $[H^+]$
PHAI	Pseudohypoaldosteronism Type 1
PHAII	Pseudohypoaldosteronism Type 2
pK	Dissociation Constant
pO_2	Oxygen Partial Pressure
PRTA	Proximal Renal Tubular Acidosis
RAAS	Renin-Angiotensin-Aldosterone System
R-Ag II	Angiotensin II Receptor
RANK	Nuclear Activator Receptor κ-B
Rhgc, Rhbg	Rhesus Glycoproteins
ROMK	Rat-Outer-Medullary K^+ Channel
RTA	Renal Tubular Acidosis
S pCO_2	Coefficient of Solubility of pCO_2 in the Alveolar Membrane (mmol/l)
	Milli-moles per Liter
SGK1	Glucocorticoid Regulated Kinase 1
SLE	Systemic Lupus Erythematosus
TAL	Potassium Secretion in the Thick Ascending Limb
TBW	Total Body Water
WNK (1–4)	"With-No-Lysine" Kinases

Chapter 1
Systemic Regulation of Acid-Base Metabolism

Javier Zamora-García and Ricardo Muñoz

Introduction: Evolutionary Aspects of Acid-Base Metabolism

The evolution of acid-base metabolism goes back to the emergence of life in the planet, about 4 billion years ago, when climatic, temperature, pH, and other physical and chemical conditions of the oceanic floor were suitable for certain molecules, such as hydrogen, oxygen, nitrogen, and carbon to bind, and perhaps facilitated the formation of amino acid chains that could be the first step to initiate life in the planet.

This could have happened around volcanic chimneys where electrical charges favored the necessary chemical reactions to create primitive life. Scientific arguments propose that certain amino acid particles, like histidine, participated in the process of assembling polypeptide chains, with subsequent RNA formation, with the capability of self-replication. These and other speculations, without convincing scientific evidence as yet, are the framework of future promising research in the

J. Zamora-García (✉)
Division of Pediatrics, Hospital Central Norte, Servicios Medicos de Petroleos Mexicanos, Mexico City, Mexico

Faculty of Medicine, National Autonomous University of Mexico, Mexico City, Mexico

R. Muñoz
Retired from: Department of Pediatric Nephrology, Hemodialysis Unit, The Children's Hospital at Albany Medical Center, Albany, NY, USA

Retired from: Pediatric Nephrology Department, Hospital Infantil de México Federico Gómez, Mexico City, Mexico

Retired from: Research Division, Hospital Infantil de Mexico Federico Gomez, Mexico City, Mexico

Retired from: National System of Investigators, Level I, Mexico City, Mexico

Retired from: North American Pediatric Renal Transplantation Collaborative Study (NAPRTCS) Study, Woburn, MA, USA

R. Muñoz (ed.), *Renal Tubular Acidosis in Children*,
https://doi.org/10.1007/978-3-030-91940-5_1

field of life evolution on the planet. Nevertheless, the theory stating that biological phenomena are the product of evolutionary mechanisms is widely accepted.

Several pioneer researchers guided the scientific thoughts upon the theory of evolution of the species on the planet, plants, and animals as well. Some of these specimens, aquatic or terrestrial, have survived until today, providing the opportunity to develop future scientific research on the understanding of the evolution of all species, including humans.

It is worth mentioning some of the investigators that guided the initial scientific work on the theory of evolution of the species, such as Charles R. Darwin 1809–1882): On the origin of species through natural selection; or The preservation of favored races in the struggle for life; Alfred R. Wallace (1823–1913): Contributions to the Theory of Natural Selection (2ª ed). London: Macmillan & Co. 1870; 384; Claude Bernard (1813–1878): written in French (Leçons sur les phénomènes de la vie comuns aux Animaux et aux végétaux. París, Librairie Philosophique J. Vrin. 1866) and, more recently, Homer Smith, with his relevant advance research on renal physiology in animals and humans: From fish to philosopher. Boston, Little, Brown & Co. 1953).

The earliest living creatures were fungi, yeasts, possible prokaryotic cells, and bacteria. Unicellular forms simply excreted the end products of their metabolism by simple vacuolization. They used O_2 in the cellular biochemical reactions during the consumption and processing of carbohydrates and the subsequent elimination of CO_2, thus giving birth to the respiratory component of the acid-base balance.

The evolution of plants and animals occurred primarily as an adaptation to the hostile environment they inhabited, and later as an adaptation to the ever-changing environmental phenomena when the organisms moved to other locations searching for better food supplies and conditions of life. The initial basic organic functions were determined by the need to conserve water and electrolyte equilibrium, as well as osmolar regulation of the cells.

Multicellular life forms appeared 3 billion years later, about 1 billion years from now. More complex organisms needed to develop adaptive mechanisms to survive under the seawater modifications that appear during this era in the ocean depths. These primitive organisms performed more complicated functions, with the development of enzymes that help to increase the speed of biochemical reactions, as well as the emergence of cell transmembrane transport proteins, facilitating the passage of water and diverse molecules from the environment through their bi-lipid cell membranes, such as aquaporins, carbonic anhydrase, and ATPases.

Under these conditions, the organisms required excretion of the excessive amount of salts from the ocean salty water, mainly Na^+Cl^-, while simultaneously, retaining electrolyte-free water in the organism. In some species, salt-secreting glands were formed to fulfill this purpose. Rudimentary renal tubules appeared first, as a simple straight tubule, with minimal variability of the tubular epithelium, a few apical microvilli, and abundant collagen material. All this occurred when primitive multicellular organisms emerged, such as mollusks, arthropods, sponges, annelids, cordata, primitive fish, etc.

Throughout millions of years, the organisms moved from salty-seawater to brackish water and, then to clear freshwater, almost free of electrolytes. At that time, the adaptive mechanisms changed oppositely to those of the previous life in the ocean, namely, the conservation of Na^+Cl^- and the excretion of excess H_2O to avoid dilution of the body fluids. Glomeruli appeared then to excrete the electrolyte free-water excess. The main function of glomeruli consisted of the ultrafiltration of large amounts of water while retaining some molecules necessary to sustain life within the vascular space, such as proteins, albumin, macromolecules, etc. Few marine species, which never left the ocean, remained without glomeruli (a-glomerular), surviving in the same way up to the present time. The simple, straight renal tubule enlarged to retain sodium chloride [1].

Subsequently, some organisms left the aqueous environment for short periods giving birth to amphibians, batrachians, and reptiles that reached dry land during longer periods, then evolving through millions of years as birds and mammals. Under these circumstances, the need to conserve both, water and salts, the renal tubules suffered important modifications appearing in what we now know as the loop of Henle. These significant tubular changes originated the countercurrent mechanism and the appearance of enzymes and hormones, such as vasopressin, oxytocin, etc., that unfold vital physiological mechanisms, such as urine concentration and dilution, osmolar regulation, fluid and, electrolyte balance and, acid-base metabolism, increasing the chances of survival in a world with constantly changing environment [2].

Similarly, some reptiles and sea birds developed salt-secreting glands (Na^+ Cl^-), to counteract the salt excess ingested from the ocean. These glands are located around the nostrils or the anal orifices, whose cells use a transporter protein, the sodium/potassium pump, or sodium-potassium adenosine-triphosphatase (Na^+/K^+ATPase), similar to the transporter protein found in the renal tubular cells of mammals, including humans. However, these salt glands transporter proteins in the nostrils work in the opposite direction of those found in the renal tubular cells of mammals. Instead of sodium reabsorption and potassium excretion in the kidney, the sodium secreting glands of birds and some reptiles (sea iguanas) expel sodium chloride from the extracellular fluid (ECF) into the environment [3]. The complex evolutionary changes briefly described herein evolved over millions of years.

During more recent periods of evolution, the mechanisms of regulation of acid-base metabolism began to develop, in a never-ending process, up to now.

Perhaps, the metabolic component of acid-base metabolism emerged during the pre-*Cambrian* period, at the end of the *Proterozoic* and the beginning of the *Paleozoic* periods, around 450 million to 500 million years ago, due to the need to excrete nitrogenous waste products from the protein metabolism. This occurred when primitive multicellular organisms emerged, such as mollusks, arthropods, sponges, annelids, cordata, etc. [4].

Some toxic end products of nitrogen metabolism have been excreted by gills, nostrils, and anal glands, as well as by the kidneys of diverse species (fish, birds, amphibians, reptiles, and mammals), as ammonia, uric acid, and urea [5]. These end products of nitrogen metabolism also help to eliminate hydrogen ions, participating in the regulation of acid-base metabolism. These chemicals are eliminated in greater or lesser quantity, depending on the capacity and adaptation characteristics of each species. Fishes use mainly ammonia (*ammonotelic*), as the end product of protein metabolism, due to the easier excretion of this compound by the gills and its capacity to dissolve in water. The participation of the kidneys in this process is of little relevance. The H^+ATPase transporter protein is active in the gills of freshwater fish; the Na^+/H^+ family of transporters in marine fish and, in both species, the anion exchange proteins (HCO_3^-/Cl^-) are the main molecules that contribute to maintaining the pH of the ECF of most aquatic species. The respiratory component of the acid-base metabolism plays a less important activity in acid-base regulation in fish [6–8].

Even though birds and certain reptiles also excrete ammonia, they mainly resorted to the formation and excretion of uric acid (*uricotelic*) for the elimination of nitrogenous waste products and protons, with the advantage of having less toxicity over ammonia, besides that only a small amount of water is required for its elimination, thus reducing body weight and facilitating the flight of birds. Contrary to acid-base physiology in fish, the mechanisms of production and excretion of CO_2 (respiratory component) in birds is the most advanced of all vertebrates in pH regulation.

Mammals, including humans, form and excrete ammonia and uric acid, but to a lesser degree of physiological importance. Mammals also developed the respiratory component of the acid-base regulation, similar to birds. Nevertheless, the most important physiological mechanism developed for nitrogenous product excretion in mammals is mainly the formation and excretion of urea (*ureotelic*), with the advantage of having the lowest risk of toxicity. Nonetheless, urea needs a greater amount of water for renal excretion. Most relevant is the fact that urea molecules also contribute to assembling the countercurrent mechanism, together with Na^+Cl^- and water [9].

Ammonia, a final product of protein metabolism of some amino acids, such as glycine, valine, methionine, etc., is highly toxic at high concentrations. Nevertheless, ammonia excretion is an important mechanism used by different species in acid-base balance. In fish and aquatic invertebrates, ammonia is eliminated through the gills, while in mammals, including humans, is used as a buffer mechanism, increasing the renal excretion of hydrogen. In this process, new bicarbonate is formed, as an evolutionary process of adaptation of some animal species to their environment. Ammonia can also be transformed to urea in various species (sharks, amphibians, and mammals) via the urea cycle, or uric acid in birds and reptiles. Uric acid may become solid, thus reducing the amount of water loss through the final urine.

The mechanisms of renal regulation of acid-base metabolism in humans are described in the corresponding chapter.

Physical and Chemical Principles of Acid-Base Metabolism

The acid-base balance is a complex process in which various biochemical factors participate; mainly the concentration of free H^+, which indicates the degree of acidity of a buffer solution and is expressed as pH. In this process participate the respiratory component, regulated by the lungs and expressed as the partial pressure of carbon dioxide (pCO_2). The metabolic component of acid-base balance is expressed by the plasma concentration of bicarbonate [HCO_3^-], regulated by the kidneys, based on glomerular and tubular physiology. Much of the complexity of acid-base regulation occurs because these components work together in a dependent manner and are expressed with different meanings; some represent "intensity", while others indicate "quantity" of the phenomenon. Thus, pCO_2 is expressed in millimeters of mercury (mmHg) and is indicative of intensity, while the concentration of bicarbonate [HCO_3^-] is expressed in milliequivalents per liter (mEq/l) or millimoles per liter (mmol/l), meaning the amount of acid-base regulatory substances present in a buffer solution. The pH, a mathematical concept, is a measure of the electrochemical potential of protons and indicates intensity. It is expressed in logarithmic units on the base of 10 [10].

The acid-base properties of organic compounds are important in the physiology of every animal species, which, from their distribution in the organism to their metabolic endpoint, are determined by the acid or base character. Furthermore, the acidity of the medium in which they are distributed also has a determining effect on their metabolism.

The first systematization of the concepts of acid and base was elaborated by Arrhenius, who in 1897 defined an acid as a "substance that, in solution, releases hydrogen ions or protons" (H^+), while a base is a "substance that, in solution, releases hydroxyl ions (OH^-)". This nomenclature has the drawback of not assigning any participation in the environment in which they are located. For this reason, Brönsted (1923) and Lowry, almost simultaneously, proposed the nomenclature according to the acid behavior concerning substances dissolved in an aqueous medium, from which it is derived that an acid is a substance capable of yielding H^+, while a base is a substance that accepts H^+, depicted in the following formula:

$$HA \leftrightarrow H^+ + A^-$$

The symmetrical behavior going in both directions in the formula determines that, for a substance to act as an acid yielding H^+, it implies the existence of another capable of behaving as a base, simultaneously. The hydroxyl group (OH^-) is a base component of the hydroxides that are part of the minerals; therefore, accepts protons. This explains that some substances that, although they do not contain OH^- groups, behave like bases, as is the case of amines that contain a nitrogenous molecule with two unshared electrons, capable of accepting or binding H^+ ions. According to this concept, different substances, when dissolved in water have a buffer capacity, since they can behave as acids or bases while accepting or releasing protons [11, 12].

Buffer Mechanisms, pH, and pK Concepts

The acidity or alkalinity of a solution is determined by the concentration of H^+, which in the ECF of the human body is 0.0000000398 (nm/l), showing slight variations in the physiological range. This figure implies a complicated mathematical assessment in clinical practice. For this reason, Sörensen (1909) proposed an alternate logarithmic application to express the concentration of H^+ with positive numbering, which instead of using the decimal or exponential denomination uses the logarithmic transformation of the molar concentration of the protons [H^+], which was named pH.

Therefore, pH is the logarithmic representation of the concentration of hydrogen ions in a buffer solution. As a result of this transformation, the fractional numbers become positive integers. Since the equation is inverse, the higher the concentration of H^+, the lower the pH value. Nowadays, pH is the most common way to express the acidity or alkalinity of a buffer solution.

The Henderson and Hasselbach equations are derived from the concept of pH, solved as follows:

$$\mathrm{Ha} \rightarrow \mathrm{H}^+ + \mathrm{a}^- = \mathrm{Ha} \leftrightarrow \mathrm{H}^+ + \mathrm{a}^-$$

Regardless of the concentrations, the proportions of the components remain constant in an equilibrium solution:

$$\begin{aligned}
&\mathrm{K} = \left[\mathrm{a}^-\right]\left[\mathrm{H}^+\right] / [\mathrm{Ha}] \\
&\left[\mathrm{H}^+\right] = \mathrm{K}[\mathrm{Ha}] / \left[\mathrm{a}^-\right] : \text{Henderson} \\
&\mathrm{pH} : 1 / \left[\mathrm{H}^+\right] \mathrm{pH} = -\log 10\left[\mathrm{H}^+\right] \\
&-\log\left[\mathrm{H}^+\right] = -\log \mathrm{K} - \log[\mathrm{Ha}] / \left[\mathrm{a}^-\right] \\
&\mathrm{pH} = \mathrm{pK} + \log\left[\mathrm{a}^-\right] / [\mathrm{Ha}] : \text{Henderson} \quad \text{Hasselbach} \\
&\mathrm{pH} = \mathrm{pK} + \log\left[\mathrm{HCO}_3^-\right] / \left[\mathrm{H}_2\mathrm{CO}_3^-\right]
\end{aligned}$$

In the extracellular fluid (ECF) of the organism the concepts of the equations are expressed in real quantities. Because the concentration of hydrogen in this fluid space is in the order of 0.0000000398 nm/l, the following results are obtained:

$$\begin{aligned}
&\mathrm{pH} = -\log\left[\mathrm{H}^+\right] \\
&\mathrm{pH} = -\log[3.98 \times 10] \\
&\mathrm{pH} = -\log\left[3.98 - \log 10^{-8}\right] \\
&-\log 3.98 = -0.60; \\
&\log 10^{-8} : 8 \\
&\mathrm{pH} = -0.60 + 8.0 = 7.40
\end{aligned}$$

Therefore, the physiological H^+ concentration of 3.98×10^{-8} in the ECF of the human body corresponds to a pH of (7.40 ± 0.05).

On the other hand, the pK concept refers to the dissociation constant of a buffer substance, and is deduced from the terms previously mentioned:

$$K = \left[H^+\right]\left[a^-\right] / \left[Ha\right]$$
$$\left[H^+\right] = K\left[Ha\right] / \left[a\right] = \text{Henderson}$$

Therefore:

$$pH = -\log H^+$$
$$\log H^+ = -\log K - \log\left[Ha\right] / \left[a^-\right]$$
$$pH = pK + -\log\left[a\right] / \left[Ha\right] = \text{Henderson - Hasselbach}$$

Thus:

$$pH = pK + \log\left[HCO_3^-\right] = pH = pK + \log\left[HCO_3^-\right] / \left[H_2CO_3\right] \times S.pCO_2 :$$

- $[H^+]$: hydrogen ion concentration
- $[a^-]$: base concentration
- −log: negative logarithm
- pH: −log $[H^+]$: hydrogen ion concentration in a buffer solution
- pK: dissociation constant of a substance
- $[HCO_3^-]$: bicarbonate concentration
- $[H_2CO_3]$: carbonic acid concentration
- $S.pCO_2$: alveolar CO_2 solubility coefficient: 0.03
- pK + log $[HCO_3^-]$: metabolic component (24 mEq/l)
- $[H_2CO_3] \times S \times pCO_2$: respiratory component (0.03)

The concept of pK is based on the Henderson-Hasselbalch equation, which represents the law of mass action, which states that the speed of a reaction equals the product of the molar concentrations of the reactants.

An acid-base buffer is a solution that contains two or more chemical compounds and prevents intense or sudden changes in the concentration of hydrogen ions.

A buffer substance is a mixture that minimizes pH changes in a solution to which an acid or alkali is added. This substance is made up of a weak acid, accompanied by an alkaline salt with a strong base; or a weak base that is accompanied by an acid salt of a strong acid.

The maximum buffer action of a solution occurs when, adding a unit of acid, a minimal change of pH appears. At this point, half of the acid is neutral and indicates that half of the buffer has dissociated. Therefore, the pH corresponds to the pK or dissociation constant of the buffer system. Strong acids such as HCl, as well as strong bases, or inert solutions, do not have a pH.

When a buffer system dissociates at 50%, pK is equal to pH; its effectiveness is at the maximum. Accordingly, the HPO_4^{-2}/HPO_4^- damper or buffer system, with a pK of 6.80 (closer to the ECF's pH of 7.40 ± 0.05), would theoretically be the most efficient buffer, which is correct only in a closed acid-base system. However, in an open system, as occurs in the human ECF, the HCO_3^-/H_2CO_3 buffer pair, with a pK of 6.10, is more efficient due to its abundance and the ability to form CO_2, which can be eliminated through the alveoli (respiratory component), as well as H^+, that can be excreted by the kidney (metabolic component) [13].

According to the titration of acids and bases, the dissociation constants (pK) of some of the buffer systems of the ECF are shown below [14]:

- Buffer pairs and their dissociation constant (pK)
- Bicarbonate/carbonic acid ($HCO_3/H_2CO_3^-$): 6.10
- Phosphates/phosphoric acid ($H_2PO_4^-/HPO_4^{-2}$): 6.80
- Acetate/Acetic acid: 3.80
- Hydroxybutirate/B-Hydroxybutyric: 4.80
- Lactate/Lactic Acid: 3.90
- Ammonia/ammonium (NH_3/NH_4^+): 9.37

To maintain the pH within the physiological range, several modifications have been developed over time. These mechanisms are present in the body fluid compartments, with certain variations in their activity. Due to technical reasons, the ECF is the compartment best studied to date.

Buffer, compensation, and correction mechanisms of the primary disturbance of the acid-base equilibrium are called defense mechanisms of the acid-base metabolism.

A buffer mechanism works using substances capable of capturing or yielding protons or hydrogen ions (H^+), or hydroxyl groups (OH^-) in the ECF via bicarbonate (metabolic component) and CO_2 (respiratory component) buffer systems. In theory, CO_2 is not an acid, since there is no H^+ molecule to be donated. However, CO_2 behaves like an acidic compound in an open metabolic system, such as the ECF, where CO_2 becomes hydrated, to be transformed into carbonic acid in a first step, and bicarbonate and hydrogen ions in a second step of the chemical reaction, called equilibrium reaction, described below [15].

CO_2 Production and Excretion

The buffer systems are listed below in qualitative order of importance, according to the buffering proportion in an open system, such as the ECF [16].

Buffer solution:	% buffering capacity in the ECF
Total bicarbonate:	53%:
HCO_3^- in plasma:	35%
HCO_3^- in erythrocytes:	18%

Hemoglobin/oxyhemoglobin:	35%
Organic phosphates:	3%
Inorganic phosphates:	2%
Plasma proteins:	7%
Total non-bicarbonate:	47%

The role CO_2 plays in the body is only partially known. However, its involvement in oxidation-reduction reactions, the importance of numerous enzyme systems, as well as the relationship with the concentration of other intracellular and extracellular ions has been well documented. These facts, as well as the precision in detecting its variations in the organic fluids, indicate that its concentration is a fine controlled homeostatic mechanism. Under physiological conditions, the tissue production of carbonic acid is 13,000–15,000 mmol/day. Pulmonary ventilation keeps the concentration of this volatile acid in the blood and tissues within normal limits.

The CO_2 produced during the cellular biochemical reactions is removed from the cytosol and dissolved in the ECF, where it joins an H_2O molecule for its conversion into carbonic acid (hydration reaction), which is accelerated by the intracellular enzyme carbonic anhydrase (AC II). The reaction proceeds to the formation of bicarbonate and H^+ ions (dissociation reaction). Bicarbonate is transported by the systemic circulation into the lungs, where the equilibrium reaction takes place, although in the opposite direction. Thus, CO_2 is formed back to be excreted as pCO_2 via the lungs. The equilibrium reaction works by buffering the excess of CO_2, as well as hydrogen ions in the ECF, expressed as follows:

Hydration and dissociation steps during the equilibrium reaction:

$$\begin{array}{l} CO_2\left(g\right)+H_2O\rightarrow CO_2\left(d\right)+H_2O\left(CA\,II\right)\leftrightarrow H_2CO_3\leftrightarrow H^+ + HCO_3^- \\ \left(\text{hydration}\right) \qquad\qquad\qquad \left(\text{dissociation}\right) \end{array}$$

where:

- CO_2 (g): CO_2 (gas)
- CO_2 (d): dissolved CO_2
- (CA II): carbonic anhydrase II
- H_2CO_3: carbonic acid
- H^+: hydrogen ion or proton
- HCO_3^-: bicarbonate

Most of the CO_2 is transported as bicarbonate (90%) in the ECF, mainly bound to a sodium molecule (Na^++HCO_3^-), while the rest is bound to other compounds, or remains dissolved (CO_2 (d)). CO_2 is transported in the venous blood bound to reduced hemoglobin, to be exchanged instead of O_2 in the pulmonary alveoli. O_2 then circulates as oxyhemoglobin, to oxygenate the tissues. During the equilibrium reaction, the proton (H^+) binds to ECF buffers (HCO_3^-). In the kidneys, hydrogen ions bind to ammonia or titratable acid, to finally be excreted in the urine. Buffering of hydrogen ions prevents sudden changes in the pH of the EEC.

The equilibrium reaction works only in an open system such as the ECF, whereas the H^+ excess gets excreted by the kidney and the pCO_2 excess is eliminated by the lungs [17].

The pH does not represent the amount of acid present in a solution, but the amount of free H^+ in a buffer solution. Most of the free H^+ are captured by buffer systems avoiding sudden changes in the pH of a solution. This action is necessary, since significant or sudden changes in the $[H^+]$ may hinder biochemical, enzymatic, and other systemic activities, vital to sustain life [15].

Acid Production and Hydrogen Balance

The body's acid-base metabolism revolves around the production and excretion of hydrogen or protons (H^+). The proton represents the atomic unit and defines acids. It is the most abundant element in the universe and is part of most biological functions.

In the body, H^+ is produced from endogenous protein metabolism. On the other hand, when entering the Krebs cycle, carbohydrates form bicarbonate when the oxidation reaction is incomplete, whereas CO_2 and H_2O are formed as complete oxidation. The CO_2 molecules are eliminated from the body through the lungs ($CO_2 \leftrightarrow pCO_2$) and the H_2O molecules by the kidneys. Therefore, carbohydrates do not represent a major source of hydrogen production under physiological conditions.

However, during pathological situations, such as hypoxia and state of shock, carbohydrate metabolism is disrupted and excess lactic acid is generated, which clinically manifests as lactic acidosis.

Fat intake also involves oxidation processing ending in the production and elimination of CO_2 and H_2O. Fatty acid metabolism is not a source of protons under physiological conditions, either. However, the interruption of the fatty acid cycle, as occurs in prolonged fasting and diabetes mellitus, results in the accumulation of acetoacetic, β-hydroxybutyric, palmitic acid, and other fatty acids as well, which generate systemic metabolic acidosis with ketoacidosis [18].

Under physiological conditions, the main source of H^+ derives from the metabolism of proteins during the production of amino acids, mainly leucine, isoleucine, valine, methionine, and arginine. The average production of protons produced in the adult is 60 to 100 mEq daily, which is equivalent to ±1 mEq of H^+/kg of body weight.

In addition to protein intake, there is another source of H^+ production in children. Due to bone mineralization, a characteristic of growth and development at this stage, the deposition of calcium and phosphates compounds to form hydroxyapatite involves the production of protons, which must be added to the metabolism of amino acids, as expressed below:

$$\left(10\,Ca^{2+} + 4.8\,HPO_4^{-} + 1.2\,H_2PO_4^{-} + 2H_2O\right) \rightarrow \left[Ca_3\left(PO_4\right)_2\right]_3 + Ca\left(OH\right)_2 + 9.2H^{+})$$

The deposit of 1 g of calcium generates ±20 mEq of H^+. Children require about 200–250 mg of Ca^{2+} daily for growth-related bone mineralization. Therefore, in children, 4–5 mEq of H^+ are produced daily. The sum of the sources of daily H^+ production in children is 2–3 mEq/kg BW daily, a significantly higher amount compared with the adults. These hydrogen ions are immediately buffered in the ECF and subsequently excreted by the kidneys, which is the only route of protons excretion from the body [19].

Acid-Base Balance

The main purpose of acid-base metabolism is intended to regulate hydrogen ion $[H^+]$ concentration in the EEC, which results from the difference of income (production) and expense (excretion) of acids and bases. In clinical practice, the diagnosis, treatment, and evolution of acid-base disorders of the organism are based on the laboratory results of some acid-base parameters that can be measured in the blood, such as bicarbonate and carbonic acid concentration; oxyhemoglobin (HbO_2), reduced hemoglobin (also called deoxyhemoglobin) ($HHbO_2$), titratable acidity (AT), and ammonium excretion. Both types of hemoglobin, as well as pH, pCO_2, and pO_2 are expressed in mEq or mmol, values that indicate intensity. The intensity indices represent the relationship between quantities or concentrations.

The pH that results of the relationship between the above parameters are regulated simultaneously by the function of lungs and kidneys and inversely related to the severity of the acid-base imbalance.

In the presence of a primary alteration of acid-base metabolism, either metabolic or respiratory acidosis or alkalosis, the body uses defense mechanisms to counteract the alteration and avoid sudden changes in $[H^+]$ or pH. In order of appearance and speed, the defense mechanisms are buffering, compensation, and correction [20].

In short, the buffer mechanism consists of using biochemical reactions, such as the equilibrium reaction in the EEC, to minimize sudden changes in pH, which hamper cellular metabolic functions that take place only within narrow limits of pH, range 7.40 ± 0.05. Another buffer mechanism is the cation exchange between the EEC and the intracellular fluid (ICF). The ECF excess of H^+ molecules exchange for ICF K^+, or bone Ca^{2+}, in the presence of systemic metabolic acidosis. These facts may explain the presence of hyperkalemia during the initial phase of acidosis. However, hypokalemia may develop in the presence of chronic acidosis due to body depletion of potassium.

A similar situation happens when ECF H^+ molecules exchange for ICF Ca^{2+} from the bone, in the presence of chronic metabolic acidosis. This is another important reason for the effectiveness of HCO_3^- as a buffer system since its presence is abundant as calcium carbonate in the bone.

Calcium and phosphates bind to form bone deposits of hydroxyapatite. Skeletal deposits are used as buffers in the presence of acute and chronic acidosis, by transporting H^+ to the cytosol of the osteocytes in exchange for Ca^{2+} molecules that are taken from the hydroxyapatite deposits toward the ECF, to avoid abrupt pH modifications. However, there is a risk of developing short-term hypercalcemia in an acute phase of metabolic acidosis. On the other hand, hypocalcemia, bone demineralization, osteopenia, and rickets are the hallmark of chronic metabolic acidosis, as in chronic renal failure [21]. Other buffer systems will be described later.

Compensation is the presence of a secondary response mechanism of the acid-base metabolism, activating a compensatory response in an organ contrary to the organ which originated the primary alteration. For example, primary metabolic acidosis is compensated by pulmonary hyperventilation and respiratory alkalosis. Similarly, a primary respiratory alkalosis will be compensated by a secondary metabolic acidosis, as a response of the kidneys by decreasing the excretion of hydrogen ions [22].

The compensation mechanisms are derived from the Henderson-Hasselbach reaction:

$$pH : pK + \log\left[HCO_3^-\right] / \left[H_2CO_3\right] + S \times pCO_2$$

- $pK + \log [HCO_3^-]$ (metabolic component)
- $[H_2CO_3] + S$ (0.03) pCO_2 (respiratory component)
- S: coefficient of solubility of pCO_2 in the alveolar membrane: (0.03)

The compensation mechanism is to minimize pH changes in the ECF, by modifying the concentration of the metabolic component or the respiratory component in the same direction as the primary alteration. Therefore, compensation is performed by the organ opposite to the component in which the primary alteration occurred, as shown in the following examples:

(a) Metabolic component: $\downarrow HCO_3^-$ (kidney) = (primary metabolic acidosis)
(b) Respiratory component: $\downarrow pCO_2$ (lung) = (compensatory respiratory alkalosis)

(a) Metabolic component: $\uparrow HCO_3^-$ (kidney) = (primary metabolic alkalosis)
(b) Respiratory component: $\uparrow pCO_2$ (lung) = (compensatory respiratory acidosis)

where: (a): primary alteration; (b) compensatory response.

When the primary alteration is respiratory, compensation occurs at the expense of the metabolic component, the physiological compensatory mechanism occurs in the kidneys. It is worth mentioning that compensation tends to avoid sudden changes in pH, but overcompensation does not happen. Therefore, in the presence of an alteration of acid-base metabolism, it is possible to differentiate which one is the primary alteration and which one is the compensatory mechanism. Consequently, in the presence of a partially compensated primary metabolic acidosis, HCO_3^- is reduced and the pH slightly reduced. In contrast, in a fully compensated primary metabolic acidosis, the HCO_3^- blood is reduced but the blood pH is at the normal value: 7.40 ± 0.05. In the presence of metabolic or respiratory alkalosis, the pH maybe slightly elevated (partially compensated) or normal (completely compensated). Therefore, the pH is not a good index to determine the presence or absence of a primary acid-base alteration, since it can be normal, depending upon the degree of compensation. In addition to pH, it is necessary to have measurements of the concentration of HCO_3^- and pCO_2 to determine the presence of a primary alteration and the degree of compensation. The equilibrium reaction participates in the process of compensation, depicted as follows:

$$CO_2(g) \rightarrow CO_2(d) + H_2O(AC) \leftrightarrow H_2CO_3 \leftrightarrow H^+ + HCO_3^- \rightarrow ECF$$

- CO_2 (d): CO_2 dissolved in the ECF
- CO_2 (g): gaseous in the ECF
- AC II: site of presence of carbonic anhydrase II
- ECF: extracellular fluid

Correction of the primary acid-base alteration is the mechanism taking care of the disappearance of all the signs and symptoms, as well as the laboratory data, of the primary acid-base disturbance. The correction mechanism involved is the same as the component of the primary alteration. For example, a primary metabolic acidosis secondary to an acute renal failure will be corrected by the organ in charge of the metabolic component; the renal pathology disappears and organ function is restored at this time. Likewise, in the case of respiratory acidosis, the exchange of pCO_2 for O_2 is corrected when the pulmonary abnormality resolves (e.g., bronchopneumonia) [23].

Example:

$$(\text{Respiratory acidosis}: CO_2\text{retention}): \text{Lung}(\uparrow pCO_2)$$
$$\rightarrow (\text{Metabolic alkalosis}: \uparrow H^+\text{excretion}): \text{Kidney}(\uparrow \text{TA}, NH_4^+)$$

- TA: titratable acidity
- NH_4^+: ammonium

The CO_2 is produced in the tissues during cellular respiration and transported as bicarbonate (HCO_3^-)/(H_2CO_3) carbonic acid, to the ECF in a 20:1 ratio, where it is attracted to the equilibrium reaction very rapidly, due to the presence of the enzyme carbonic anhydrase, and finally excreted by the lungs. The bicarbonate/carbonic acid buffer system is quantitatively the most important in the organism, although the dissociation constant (pK 6.10) is far from the ECF pH of 7.40 ± 0.05. This fact is compensated by the abundance of bicarbonate in the ECF (24–26 mmol/l) and by the body capacity to transport CO_2 in the form of bicarbonate through the equilibrium reaction in an open buffer system, as it happens in the ECF. This buffering pair works in an open system with the ability to remove CO_2 from the lungs as partial pressure (pCO_2) in the gas mixture found in an alveolar air, which is similar to the mixture of gases in the atmosphere we breathe. The total atmospheric pressure is 760 mmHg at sea level, at 25 °C of environmental temperature [24]. The total atmospheric pressure of a mixture of gas is the result of the partial pressure of each gas that makes up the mixture, the percentage of which is shown below:

- Nitrogen: 68%
- Oxygen: 20%
- Carbon dioxide: 5%
- Water vapor: 7%

The partial pressure of each gas is deduced from the pressure of the total mixture. For example, CO_2: 5% (.05) × 760 mmHg: pCO_2: 38 mmHg (±40 mmHg, as standardized in clinical routine practice) [25].

Hemoglobin and Erythrocyte Physiology

The second buffering system of acid-base metabolism, in order of importance, is limited to the circulatory system and refers to the oxyhemoglobin/deoxyhemoglobin (HbO_2/Hb) buffer system. The latter is also called reduced hemoglobin. During the respiratory process, when excreting pCO_2 by the alveolar exchange for O_2 (in the ferric group of hemoglobin), one H^+ molecule is captured in the imidazole group. On the contrary, during cellular respiration, hemoglobin transfers the O_2 molecule to the cytosol in exchange for CO_2, and the imidazole group captures an H^+ molecule to form reduced hemoglobin, which is why the HbO_2/Hb system is important as a buffering mechanism during the process of systemic regulation of acid-base metabolism (Fig. 1.1).

In the circulatory system, the concentration of oxyhemoglobin in arterial blood is 95%, while that of reduced hemoglobin is 5%. In venous blood, reduced hemoglobin concentration is 75% and oxyhemoglobin 25%.

The molecular structure of hemoglobin bound to globin belongs to the heme group and consists of an imidazole group, with 2 nitrogen molecules, $2H^+$ (HN-HN), and 2 carbon (C) molecules that bind to a ferric group by a nitrogen molecule. The iron group carries O_2 from the lungs to the tissues, and the acid-base buffering occurs in the imidazole group. Oxygen is captured in the alveolar wall in exchange for a CO_2 molecule, which is excreted by the lungs as pCO_2.

An H^+ ion becomes detached from the imidazole group during the capture of O_2 by the ferric group, while an H^+ is detached from the imidazole group and diffuses into the plasma for its buffering by bicarbonate.

O_2 is transported in the red cells through the circulatory system to the capillaries located in tissues, then to the cellular mitochondria to generate the necessary energy in all cells of the body. The opposite phenomenon happens in the tissues, where O_2 is bound to the iron group of hemoglobin to be delivered to the cells, which in turn releases a CO_2 molecule. In the process, an H^+ molecule is captured and the buffering circle in the ECF is completed.

The CO_2 produced during cellular respiration is transported by the systemic circulation and eliminated through the alveolar capillaries. The transport of dissolved

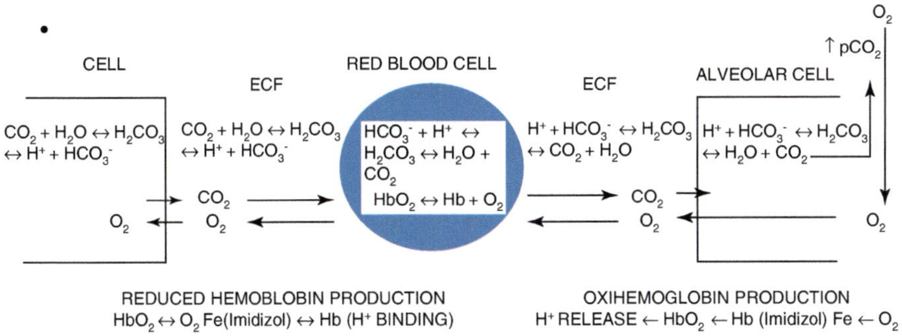

Fig. 1.1 Bicarbonate-hemoglobin buffer systemic transport. The CO_2 produced on the tissues gets transported to the extracellular fluid space (ECF), where bicarbonate (HCO_3^-) is made via the equilibrium reaction, which is the main form of CO_2 transport in the ECF. Small amounts are transported as dissolved carbon dioxide (CO_2) and carbonic acid (H_2CO_3). HCO_3^- is captured by the red blood cell, where is transported to the pulmonary alveoli until its final excretion from the lungs as pCO_2 (partial pressure of CO_2), in exchange for O_2. During this process, reduced hemoglobin (Hb) is produced in the red blood cell, where an H^+ molecule is captured. The O_2 molecules captured in the lungs are transported toward the opposite direction, firstly to the ECF, and red blood cells where they bind to the ferric group (Fe^{++}) of imidazole at the reduced hemoglobin (Hb), to be transformed into oxyhemoglobin (HbO_2), also called saturated hemoglobin, and the final release of O_2 to the tissues, in exchange for CO_2. During oxyhemoglobin production, a molecule of H^+ is released. CO_2 is transported in the RBC, together with the reduced hemoglobin to form carbaminohemoglobin ($HbCO_2$). During the oxygenation of the tissues and the simultaneous excretion of CO_2, the buffering mechanisms HCO_3^-/H_2CO_3 and Hb/HbO_2 overlap, being the most important buffering mechanisms involved in the systemic balance of acid-base metabolism, because of the capture and release of hydrogen ions

CO_2 in the ECF, plasma, erythrocytes, and the alveolar membrane is facilitated by the equilibrium reaction, in the presence of the enzyme intracellular carbonic anhydrase (AC II). Because cellular CO_2 is produced in the cells at a faster pace than the lung clearance, the equilibrium reaction also takes place in the ECF, where CO_2 is converted to carbonic acid and bicarbonate, being this the most abundant form of CO_2 transport. In the plasma fluid, the main buffers are bicarbonate/carbonic acid and plasma proteins [17, 26].

On the other hand, in the erythrocyte, the carbonic acid/bicarbonate and oxyhemoglobin/reduced hemoglobin systems prevail, favored by the presence of carbonic anhydrase and some of the aquaporins, which transport H_2O molecules into the erythrocyte, which is the substrate for the intracellular equilibrium reaction.

Another important factor that contributes to the process is the anionic antitransporter (AE1), which performs the exchange of plasma chloride (Cl^-) for HCO_3^- in the erythrocyte. Molecules of HCO_{3-} from the erythrocyte become part of the buffering process, both in plasma and in the rest of the ECF. The erythrocyte plays an important role in the buffering process by these systems [27–29].

The phosphate/phosphoric acid buffer system is of no quantitative importance at the systemic level but becomes relevant during the renal excretion of hydrogen in the form of titratable acidity, which will be discussed together with the ammonia/ammonium system in the corresponding chapter.

Clinical Aspects of Alterations in Acid-Base Metabolism

Variations of the pH in the ECF occur when free hydrogen ion concentrations are altered. Increased [H^+] concentration leads to acidosis; with a pH of <7.35. On the contrary, metabolic alkalosis develops when [H^+] decreases and pH increases to >7.45. This clinical nomenclature is used to describe alterations of acid-base metabolism and the diagnosis of the primary metabolic alteration. The mechanisms of buffering and compensation may also be supported by the blood gas determinations. Therefore, metabolic acidosis is the disorder characterized by the accumulation of hydrogen ions, or by the loss of bases, mainly bicarbonate from the EEC. Metabolic alkalosis is the opposite situation, meaning the loss of hydrogen ion, or the gain of bases, referring mainly to bicarbonate of the EEC.

In contrast, respiratory acidosis means the accumulation of pCO_2 and respiratory alkalosis refers to the reduction of pCO_2 from EEC, as a result, CO_2 accumulation or losses via the lungs.

This terminology is used as a physiological clinical guide to determine the etiology of the primary alteration, as well as the presence and degree of the compensatory mechanisms involved in a clinical situation.

Disorders of acid-base balance depend on the depletion or excess of bicarbonate or hydrogen ion (metabolic component), as well as the excess or depletion of carbonic acid, converted to pCO_2 (respiratory component).

It is important to differentiate the simple from the mixed alterations of the acid-base balance. The latter has two primary acid-base alterations that affect directly both components (metabolic or respiratory) at the same time, a situation that hinders the mechanisms of compensation. It also increases the degree of difficulty in the understanding of the clinical entity and its diagnosis [30].

According to the Henderson–Hasselbach equation, blood pH is determined by the balance (20:1 ratio) between the metabolic component (plasma bicarbonate), which is corrected by the kidneys and the respiratory component (plasma pCO_2), corrected by the lungs.

A simple alteration of the acid-base balance is observed when one of the components is affected primarily, with or without a compensatory response [31].

To diagnose the type of acid-base disorder and the presence or absence of some degree of compensation, it is necessary to determine the arterial blood gases, which should be interpreted according to the normal values at different ages. Venous blood gas determination is used at some places since the difference between arterial and venous blood results is not wide. Nonetheless, arterial blood samples are of the utmost importance when the initial diagnosis is intended, leaving the venous blood samples for follow-up during stable clinical situations. The venous blood must be collected without the use of a tourniquet and preferably, arterialized venous blood. To do so, it is necessary to warm to the arm with an electric device or warm water, for few minutes, avoiding burns. This will be evaluated in the corresponding chapter on the diagnosis of renal tubular acidosis [17].

Metabolic Acidosis

This is the most frequent disorder of acid-base balance in pediatrics, mostly seen in clinical entities leading to the gain of acids or the loss of bicarbonate from the ECF. The etiology may be associated with renal or extra-renal pathology. In children, it is frequently associated with the loss of fluids and HCO_3^- from the ECF by intestinal losses, such as diarrhea, and less frequently due to an intestinal fistula, ileostomy, etc. Diarrhea is one of the main causes of metabolic acidosis, due to a high bicarbonate concentration in the intestinal secretions (80 mEq/l). Another route of HCO_3^- losses is by the kidneys, as it happens in renal tubular acidosis or during treatment with the diuretic acetazolamide, which inhibits the enzyme carbonic anhydrase, with a consequent renal tubular loss of sodium bicarbonate secondary to the blocking of the equilibrium reaction [32–35].

The second possible mechanism for the development of metabolic acidosis is the gain of hydrogen in ECF, during various clinical entities in which endogenous or exogenous acids compounds are added to the ECF, including acute or chronic renal failure, diabetic ketoacidosis, lactic acidosis, diseases of the intermediate metabolism, etc. In renal failure, phosphoric and sulfuric acids are retained during renal failure; fatty acids such as acetoacetic acid, β-hydroxybutyric acids, and so on, are also gained in diabetic ketoacidosis; whereas in lactic acidosis the gain of H^+ is as lactic acid; and in methylmalonic acidosis, the acid with the same name is retained. Retention of acids by the exogenous route may include the administration of ammonium chloride; salicylic acid, etc.

The increased H^+ load during these clinical situations consumes bicarbonate that is normally used in the buffering process of the ECF [36, 37].

Clinical observation of the patient is the most important step to find the etiology of acid-base alterations, e.g., the presence of diarrhea or vomiting, diabetic ketoacidosis, dehydration, drug ingestion, etc. The laboratory results (blood gases, serum and urine electrolytes, serum creatinine, etc.) support the diagnosis of the alteration, as well as the degree of compensation. Compensation for a primary impairment of acid-base metabolism is carried out by the organ contrary to that of the primary impairment so that in metabolic acidosis the compensation is performed by the lungs and a compensatory respiratory alkalosis develops. In the presence of a primary metabolic alkalosis, compensatory respiratory acidosis develops.

On the other hand, during respiratory acidosis the compensation is carried out by the kidneys, losing H^+ ions and retaining HCO_3^-; consequently, a metabolic alkalosis develops. During respiratory alkalosis, the compensatory renal mechanism consists of H^+ ions retention (metabolic acidosis).

Analysis of blood gases in metabolic acidosis shows a reduction in $[HCO_3^-]$, compared to the normal values for the patient's age. Plasma HCO_3^- concentration in the pediatric age group ranges at 16–26 mmol/l [38]. However, the pH may be in or out of the normal range, since the pH is independent of the actual $[H^+]$ and $[HCO_3^-]$. Instead, it depends on the proportions between both components, depending on the degree of buffering and compensation of the primary alteration.

In cases of primary metabolic acidosis, the compensatory response belongs to the lungs, with the development of hyperventilation and compensatory respiratory alkalosis. When the pH is below <7.35 and the pCO_2 is within the normal range (38–40 mmHg), it indicates that there is no adequate respiratory compensation response. Therefore, the alteration is a decompensated metabolic acidosis.

If the pH is reduced, but the pCO_2 shows only a slight or moderate reduction, the alteration is a partially compensated metabolic acidosis. If the pCO_2 becomes more reduced, meaning a good compensatory response, the pH will be within the normal range, indicating a fully compensated metabolic acidosis [39]. During a complete compensation, the pH is normal, but within the lowest normal range values.

It is important to mention that an over-compensatory effect does not take place under any circumstances. Therefore, in the presence of metabolic acidosis, with reduced plasma $[HCO_3^-]$, the pH will be reduced if no compensation or only an incomplete compensation is present. On the other hand, the pH will be normal (toward the minimal normal range) and the pCO_2 appears very low, a complete compensated metabolic acidosis is present. Thus, in this case, the compensatory response is a respiratory alkalosis.

Therefore, under these considerations, the pH is not a reliable index to establish the diagnosis of the primary alteration, since it may show normal, reduced, or high values. This is the reason pH is not considered in the definition of acid-base metabolism disorders. Instead, the pH value becomes very important to assess the degree of compensation achieved in the presence of an acid-base alteration.

The presence of mixed alterations of acid-base metabolism makes more complicated the interpretation of the laboratory results. For example, in the case of a primary metabolic acidosis, with reduced $[HCO_3^-]$, which happens to occur with a simultaneous primary respiratory alkalosis (with a reduction of pCO_2), the pH is increased if the degree of respiratory alkalosis predominates over metabolic acidosis. The 95% confidence limit curves facilitate the diagnosis of the degree of compensation, either acutely or chronically, present in an individual, for both primary and mixed disorders of the acid-base metabolism [40].

The acid-base normal lab values for the pediatric age group differ from those of the adult population. An over-diagnosis of renal tubular acidosis in children has been seen during the last decade in some Latin American countries.

This happens when the adult lab values are taken as a reference, instead of the pediatric lab values according to the patient's age, leading to an erroneous diagnosis of RTA. The sample to measure blood gases must be taken from an artery, preferentially or from a venous source, after warming the extremity, without the use of a tourniquet [41, 42]. Besides, it is convenient to consider the altitude above sea level when living in high altitude places, since all these confounding factors modify the blood gas results [43].

Correction of the primary alteration is, in chronological order, the last defense mechanism of the acid-base metabolism. However, its importance becomes obvious, since this mechanism fully corrects the primary acid-base alteration. The correction mechanism works in the metabolic component where the primary alteration appears. Thus, the kidneys correct the metabolic component and the lungs correct the respiratory component. This occurs when the etiology producing the alteration, either endogenous or exogenous, disappears spontaneously, or after treatment.

Metabolic Alkalosis

This alteration of the acid-base balance results from the gain of bicarbonate or the loss of hydrogen ions from the EEC. Clinical entities that result from the gain of bicarbonate are often iatrogenic, such as excessive administration of alkaline solutions, or prolonged use of diuretics, steroids, and antacids (sodium bicarbonate).

H^+ depletion develops by vomiting or upper intestinal obstruction, as hydrochloric acid loss, as in cases with congenital pyloric stenosis. Other causes include cystic fibrosis of the pancreas (with chloride losses); excess mineralocorticoid states, with K^+ depletion; primary and secondary hyperaldosteronism; Bartter's disease; some types of neoplasia (with hypercalcemia), etc. [32, 44].

Most cases of bicarbonate retention have none or few clinical manifestations, except in severe cases of alkalosis, with decompensation and very alkaline serum pH, when neurological manifestations appear, due to cerebral edema or hypotonia, as well as cardiac arrhythmias secondary to severe hypokalemia [45].

The compensation mechanism is mainly hypoventilation, with pulmonary CO_2 retention and increased pCO_2 to reduce the blood pH (compensatory respiratory acidosis). Also, the pH increase leads to inhibition of the respiratory center, which decreases pulmonary ventilation, with increased pCO_2 in the process of restoration of the HCO_3^-/H_2CO_3 ratio of 20:1.

Initial laboratory results show an increase [HCO_3^-] and pH as well. However, while the compensation mechanism advances, a progressive compensatory increase in pCO_2 is observed, decreasing the plasma pH. Thus, a partially compensated respiratory acidosis ensues. Complete compensation occurs after reducing plasma pH to normal levels [46].

The correction mechanism occurs when the disease or clinical situation that caused the metabolic alkalosis disappears. Metabolic alkalosis is corrected by the kidneys, by excreting bicarbonate and reabsorbing hydrogen ions in the β-intercalated cells of the collector ducts in the distal nephron.

However, in the presence of dehydration (loss of Na^+Cl^- and H_2O) and hypokalemia (loss of potassium through vomiting), β-intercalated cells in renal collecting tubules fail to excrete bicarbonate as $K^+HCO_3^-$, in exchange H^+, as it should be doing to correct the alkalosis. There is still controversy over the physiological mechanism to explain such an event. Apparently, during a primary metabolic alkalosis with fluid volume deficit, and ECF and ICF potassium depletion, Na^+Cl^- molecules compete for the sites of H^+ and K^+ reabsorption. Therefore, persistent dehydration and hypokalemia hinder the kidneys to perform the correction of alkalosis, thus, acid urine production will continue ("paradoxical aciduria") [47].

During the presence of primary metabolic acidosis or alkalosis, the pulmonary compensation response occurs rapidly. As an example, tachypnea and deep respirations appear within minutes after the presence of the primary metabolic alteration. On the other hand, during primary respiratory disorders, acidosis or alkalosis, the renal compensatory mechanism develops slowly, taking hours or days for the maximum response to develop. However, the degree of compensation achieved by the renal response is greater than the respiratory compensation.

Respiratory Acidosis

Respiratory acidosis is the clinical condition characterized by CO_2 retention with an increase in pCO_2, accompanied or not, by a plasma pH <7.35, depending on the presence or absence of the compensation mechanism.

Plasma pCO_2 may suffer faster changes than the other acid-base balance variables, such as bicarbonate or pH. During primary CO_2 retention, the pCO_2 is increased as a result of alveolar hypoventilation. The main causes of hypoventilation are disturbances of the respiratory center, such as the use of narcotics, sedatives, traumatic brain injury, encephalitis; bronchopulmonary disorders, such as bronchiolitis, bronchopneumonia, airway obstruction, pneumothorax, hemothorax, emphysema, bronchial asthma, as well as chest wall anomalies, poliomyelitis, *myasthenia gravis*, congenital malformations or trauma to the rib cage, among others.

As already mentioned, the compensation mechanism is carried out by the body fluids in the opposite direction of that of the primary alteration. When pulmonary ventilation is altered, a primary respiratory acidosis ensues and the compensation mechanism is carried out by the kidneys, which increases the excretion of H^+ ions and HCO_3^- reabsorption, mainly in the α-intercalated cells of the collecting tubules. A compensatory metabolic alkalosis appears.

Correction of the primary disorder occurs when the pCO_2 excess is eliminated, once the normal respiratory function is restored [48].

Respiratory Alkalosis

Respiratory alkalosis occurs as a result of sustained hyperventilation, leading to a decrease in pCO_2, in the presence or absence of changes in the plasma pH, again, depending on the presence and degree of compensation. Respiratory alkalosis is described in association with various pathological states, such as psychological or emotional situations accompanied by anxiety or prolonged crying with hyperventilation, all ending in pCO_2 reduction. It also occurs frequently during anesthesia, in respiratory ailments, the use of some medications, intense exercise, traumatic brain injury, etc.

Compensation is done by the kidneys, which increase the excretion of HCO_3^- and the reabsorption of H^+ in the β-intercalated cells of the collecting tubules, rendering a compensatory metabolic acidosis.

The correction of the primary acid-base alteration is carried out by the lungs when the disease or clinical etiological situation subsides and pulmonary hyperventilation ceases.

As previously mentioned, the physiological definition of acid-base disorders is based on the value of the $[HCO_3^-]_s$, which is reduced in acidosis and increased in alkalosis, respectively. A similar situation occurs in primary respiratory disorders in which the pCO_2 value determines the type of alteration, being increased in acidosis and decreased in alkalosis.

In the presence of a primary alteration of acid-base metabolism, the pH can be normal, low or, high, depending on the presence or absence of the compensation mechanism, and its degree. Therefore, the low or high pH indicates the presence of acidosis or alkalosis but does not provide precise information regarding the type of acid-base disorder [44].

Mixed Acid-Base Alterations

Mixed disorders of acid-base metabolism are the simultaneous presence of two primary disorders, in any possible combination of the four clinical disorders described above. Both alterations exert an antagonistic effect upon each other, becoming a clinical diagnostic challenge.

In general terms, the etiology is independent of each alteration. The clinical presentation dictates the type of combination of the mixed alterations. The lab results show a mixture of both alterations, with no presence of a compensatory response. These confusing lab results may be mistakenly interpreted as overcompensation. However, the physiological phenomenon of overcompensation does not happen during the regulation of the acid-base metabolism.

In mixed alterations, the pH result is erratic, it can be normal, increased, or decreased, depending on the alteration prevailing at a certain time. For example, a primary metabolic acidosis due to an acute kidney failure can occur simultaneously with a primary respiratory alkalosis during a concomitant lung disease. The laboratory results, although erratic during the initial phase of the alteration, change as the evolution of the clinical case progresses. It may show reduced HCO_3^- (metabolic acidosis) with a pCO_2 also reduced (respiratory alkalosis). In this case, the pH may be decreased, normal, or increased, which depends on the predominantly mixed alteration at the time of taking the sample for the blood gas determination.

Another example can occur when respiratory alkalosis and metabolic alkalosis occur simultaneously, the lab results show increased pCO_2 and HCO_3^-, with no evidence of compensation. The pH is higher than that assumed for a primary alteration without concomitant mixed alteration, during which the compensatory mechanism appears. A clinical example could be the patient who presents with severe vomiting and significant loss of $H^{+}Cl^{-}$ (metabolic alkalosis), with hyperventilation due to a concomitant pulmonary alteration (respiratory alkalosis) [49].

The nomograms of the primary disturbances of acid-base metabolism and the maximum degree of compensation that can be achieved may help to make the differential diagnosis of a primary disorder with adequate compensation versus mixed disturbances of acid-base metabolism [21].

References

1. Schmidt-Nielsen BM, Nissenson AR, Mackay WC. Chapter 2: Comparative physiology of electrolyte and water regulation, with emphasis on sodium, potassium, chloride, urea, and osmotic pressure. In: Maxwell MH, Kleeman CR, editors. Clinical disorders of fluid and electrolyte metabolism. 3rd ed. New York: McGraw-Hill; 1980. p. 37–88.
2. Pitts RF. Mechanisms of reabsorption and excretion of ions and water. In: Physiology of the kidney and body fluids. Chicago: Year Book Medical Publishers Inc.; 1963. p. 91–115.
3. Reineck HJ, Stein JH. Regulation of sodium balance. In: Maxwell MH, Kleeman CR, editors. Clinical disorders of fluid and electrolyte metabolism. 3rd ed. New York: McGraw-Hill Book, Co.; 1980. p. 89–111.
4. Schmith-Nielsen K. The salt-secreting glands of marine birds. Circulation. 1960;21(5):955–67.
5. Wright PA. Nitrogen excretion: three end products, many physiological roles. J Exp Biol. 1995;198:273–81.
6. Randall DJ, Tsui TKN. Tribute to RG Boutilier: acid-base transfer across fish gills. J Exp Biol. 2006:1179–84.
7. Perry SF, Shahsarvrani A, Gerorgalis T. Channels, pumps, and exchangers in the gill and kidney of freshwater fishes: their role in ionic and acid-base regulation. J Exp Zool A Comp Exp Biol. 2013;300(1):53–62.
8. Sullivan GV, Perry SF. Localization of mRNA for the proton pump (H^{+}ATPase) and exchanger in the rainbow trout gill. Can J Zool. 1996;74:20195–2013.
9. McNabb RA, McNabb FM. Urate excretion by the avian kidney. Comp Biochem Physiol A Comp Physiol. 1975;51(2):253–8.
10. Gordillo PG. Balance Ácido Base. In: Electrolitos en Pediatría Fisiología y Clínica. 3rd ed. México: Ediciones Médicas del Hospital Infantil de México; 1983. p. 155–75.
11. Petrucci RH, Harwood WS. Ácidos y bases. In: Química general. 8ª ed. Madrid: Prentice Hall; 2003. p. 665–710.
12. Petrucci RH, Harwood WS. Otros aspectos del equilibrio acido-base. In: Quimica general. 8ª ed. Madrid: Prentice Hall; 2003. p. 710–49.
13. Kennelly PJ, Rodwell VW, Agua y pH. In: Murray RK, Bender DA, editors. Harper Bioquimica Illustrada. 29ª ed. China: McGraw Hill; 2012. p. 7–15.
14. Halperin ML, Goldstein MB. Fluid, electrolyte, and acid-base emergencies. Philadelphia: Saunders; 1988. p. 2–119.
15. Mc Namara J, Worthley LIG. Acid-base balance: part I physiology. Crit Care Resusc. 2001;3:117–62.
16. Dell RB. Normal acid-base regulation. In: Winters RW, editor. The body fluids in pediatrics. 1st ed. Boston: Little Brown Co.; 1973. p. 23–45.
17. Guyton WF, Hall JE. Regulación del Equilibrio Acido-base. In: Tratado de Fisiología Medica. 12ª ed. Madrid: Elsevier; 2011. p. 484–94.

18. Carl GM, Tobin JR, Metabolic and endocrine disease in pediatric intensive care. In: Rogers MC, editor. Textbook of pediatric intensive care, vol I, 2nd ed. Baltimore: Williams and Wilkins; 1992. p. 1235–83.
19. Portale AA. Calcium and phosphorus. In: Avner ED, Harmon WE, Niaudet P, editors. Pediatric nephrology. 5th ed. Philadelphia: Lippincott Williams & Wilkins; 2004. p. 209–36.
20. Koeppen BM. Renal regulation of acid-base balance. Adv Physiol Educ. 1998;20:132–41.
21. Chan JCM, Mak RHK. Acid-base homeostasis. In: Avner ED, Harmon WE, Niaudet P, editors. Pediatric nephrology. 5th ed. Philadelphia: Lippincott Williams & Wilkins; 2004. p. 189–208.
22. Adelman RD, Solhung MJ. Fisiopatología de los líquidos corporales y tratamiento con líquidos, hidrogeniones. In: Behrman RE, Kliegman RM, Arvin AM, editors. Tratado de Pediatría, vol I. Madrid: MaGraw Hill; 1997. p. 229–72.
23. Marshall WJ, Bangert SK, Lapsley ML. Hydrogen ion homeostasis and blood gases. In: Marshall WJ, Bangert SK, Lapsley ML, editors. Clinical chemistry. 7th ed. Edinburgh: Mosby; 2012. p. 41–62.
24. Hamilton PK, Morgan NA, Connolly GM, Alexander P, Maxwell AP. Understanding acid-base disorders. Ulster Med J. 2017;86(3):161–6.
25. Winters RW, Mag KE, Dell RB. Acid-base physiology in medicine. 2nd ed. Ontario: The London Co.; 1969.
26. Winters RW, Engel K, Dell RB. The respiratory component of acid-base equilibrium. In: Winters RW, Engel K, Dell RB, editors. Acid-base physiology in medicine. 2nd ed. Cleveland: The London Co.; 1967. p. 69–94.
27. Perutz MF. Molecular anatomy, physiology, and pathology of hemoglobin. In: Stamatoyannopoulos G, Nienhuis AW, editors. The molecular basis of blood disorders. Philadelphia: WB Saunders; 1987. p. 127.
28. Wu F, Satchwell TJ, Toye AM. Anion exchanger 1 in red blood cells and kidney: band 3's in a pod. Biochem Cell Biol. 2011;89(2):106–14.
29. Blank ME, Ehmke H. Aquaporin-1 and HCO_3^--Cl^-transporter-mediated transport of CO_2 across the human erythrocyte membrane. https://doi.org/10.1113/jphysiol.2003.040113.
30. Narins RG, Emmett M. Simple and mixed acid-base disorders: a practical approach. Baltimore: Medicine; 1980. p. 59–161.
31. Kellum JA. Disorders of acid-base balance. Crit Care Med. 2007;35:2630–6.
32. Pan CG. Metabolic acid-base disturbances. In: Kher KK, Makker SP, editors. Clinical pediatric nephrology. Ed. McGraw-Hill; 1992. p. 643–63.
33. Seiter I. Integration of acid-base and electrolyte disorders. N Engl J Med. 2014;371:1821–31.
34. Finberg L. Diarrheal dehydration. In: Winters RW, editor. The body fluids in pediatrics. Boston: Little Brown Co.; 1973. p. 349–371.
35. Muñoz AR, Escobar L, Medeiros M. Acidosis tubular renal en niños: conceptos actuales de diagnóstico y tratamiento. Bol Med Hosp Infant Mex. 2013;70(3):178–94.
36. Finkel KW, DuBose TD. Metabolic acidosis. In: DuBose TD, Hamm LL, editors. Acid-base and electrolyte disorders. Philadelphia: Saunders; 2002. p. 55–66.
37. Dell RB. Diabetic ketoacidosis. In: Winters RW, editor. The body fluids in pediatrics. Boston: Little Brown Co.; 1973. p. 372–84.
38. Custer JW. Blood chemistries and body fluids. In: Custer JW, Rau RE, editors. The Harriet Lane handbook. 18th ed. Philadelphia: Mosby; 2009. p. 677–88.
39. Fulop M. A guide for predicting arterial CO2 tension in metabolic acidosis. Am J Nephrol. 1997;17(5):421.
40. Winters RW, Knud E, Dell RB. Acid-Base physiology in medicine. 2nd ed. The London Company: Cleveland; 1969.
41. Muñoz AR, Escobar L, Medeiros M. Sobre-diagnóstico de acidosis tubular renal en México. Rev Investig Clin. 2012;64:399–401.
42. Vázquez García C, Pérez Padilla R. Rev Inst Nal Enf Resp Mex. 2000;(13):6–13.
43. Tinoco AS, Angie Román Santamaría AR, Charri VJ. Gasometría arterial en diferentes niveles de altitud en residentes adultos sanos en el Perú. Horizonte Médico. 2017;(17):6–10.

44. Galla JH. Metabolic alkalosis. In: DuBose TD, Hamm LL, editors. Acid-base and electrolyte disorders. Philadelphia: Saunders; 2002. p. 109–28.
45. Taylor ND, Cass DT, Holland AJ. Infantile hypertrophic pyloric stenosis: has anything changed? J Paediatr Child Health. 2013;49:33.
46. Winters RW. Metabolic alkalosis of pyloric stenosis. In: Winters RW, editor. The body fluids in pediatrics. Boston: Little Brown Co.; 1973. p. 402–414.
47. Halperin ML, Kamel KS, Goldstein MB. Respiratory acid-base disturbances. In: Halperin ML, Kamel KS, Goldstein MB, editors. Fluid, electrolyte, and acid-base physiology. Toronto: Saunders; 2010. p. 222–42.
48. Walmsley R, White NGH. Mixed acid-base disorders. Clin Chem. 1985:321–5.
49. Brouhard BH, Cunningham III RJ, Lynch RE, Travis LB. Special problems of electrolyte, water, and acid-base metabolism in children. In: Chan JCM, Gill JR, editors. Kidney electrolyte disorders. New York: Churchill Livingstone; 1990. p. 421–56.

Chapter 2
Renal Regulation of Acid-Base Metabolism

Ricardo Muñoz

Introduction

As mentioned in the previous chapter, the lungs perform the task of removing organic volatile acids in the form of pCO_2, in exchange for oxygen. The kidneys eliminate non-volatile organic acids that contain hydrogen (protons), which includes H^+ from the intermediate metabolism, by which the dietary proteins participating in the formation of amino acids, such as leucine, isoleucine, valine, arginine, and methionine, are metabolized. Most of the H^+ is excreted as buffer systems to be excreted into the urine. One such system, "titratable acid" (TA), is composed of the buffer pairs phosphoric acid/phosphates and sulfuric acid/sulfates. The other system is composed of ammonium/ammonia [1].

The excretion of hydrogen ions or protons and, in consequence, the formation of bicarbonate, depends on several factors, such as the glomerular filtration rate; the systemic pH (influencing H^+ excretion along the nephron); the apical (luminal) pH; intracellular pH; concentration of HCO_3^- and the peritubular pCO_2, as well as the action exerted by angiotensin II (Ag II) upon proximal reabsorption of Na^+.

The renal tubular excretion of hydrogen ions is coupled to the excretion and reabsorption of sodium. Therefore, some physiological mechanisms that affect the renal handling of sodium will also affect the renal regulation of acid-base

R. Muñoz (✉)
Retired from: Department of Pediatric Nephrology, Hemodialysis Unit, The Children's Hospital at Albany Medical Center, Albany, NY, USA

Retired from: Pediatric Nephrology Department, Hospital Infantil de México Federico Gómez, Mexico City, Mexico

Retired from: Research Division, Hospital Infantil de Mexico Federico Gomez, Mexico City, Mexico

Retired from: North American Pediatric Renal Transplantation Collaborative Study (NAPRTCS) Study, Woburn, MA, USA

R. Muñoz (ed.), *Renal Tubular Acidosis in Children*,
https://doi.org/10.1007/978-3-030-91940-5_2

metabolism, being mainly the electrolyte composition and volume of the extracellular fluid (ECF); enzymatic and hormonal substances; transmembrane transport proteins; concentration gradient difference between the apical membranes of the renal tubular cell cytoplasm and luminal fluid, as well as between the cytoplasm and the peritubular fluid across the basolateral membrane [2]. Some of these mechanisms will be described below.

Hydrogen Excretion and Bicarbonate Reabsorption in the Proximal Tubule

The main function of the proximal tubule is the reabsorption of sodium chloride and other electrolytes, water, bicarbonate, glucose, calcium, magnesium, phosphates, sulfates, and small amounts of some amino acids and other chemicals filtered by the glomeruli. Most of these substances are recovered by the proximal tubules, through reabsorption in the three segments, S1, S2, and S3.

The proximal tubule's main function regarding acid-base metabolism is the excretion of hydrogen ions and reabsorption of bicarbonate. The amount of H^+ excreted by the kidneys is about 4200 mmol daily, in an adult subject with normal renal function. Most of the filtered bicarbonate is reabsorbed in the proximal tubules. Hydrogen ion excretion is accomplished by the production and excretion of TA and ammonia. The buffer pair ammonium/ammonia is produced mainly, but not exclusively, in the proximal tubule. The main area of excretion of ammonia is the final portion of the nephron, as will be described in the next section.

Some buffer substances within the ECF also undergo glomerular filtration. Bicarbonate, which is the main ECF buffer, is filtered as sodium bicarbonate. The apical membranes of the proximal tubular cells cannot reabsorb $NaHCO_3$ molecules as such. Therefore, this molecule dissociates as Na^+ and HCO_3^- molecules in the proximal luminal fluid. The Na^+ molecule gets reabsorbed in the apical (luminal) membrane of the brush border cells by the action of several mechanisms, mainly a transmembrane transporter protein sodium/hydrogen exchanger (Na^+/H^+), named NHE3, in an electroneutral exchange. Several NHE3 isoforms function on both the apical and basolateral membranes, depending on the physiological need of each site [3–6] (Fig. 2.1). Furthermore, the Na^+ molecules are reabsorbed through Na^+ channels, or by coupling with other molecules, such as glucose, phosphates, sulfates, amino acids, citrates, and other organic acids [7]. The proximal sodium reabsorption process ends up in the basolateral membrane by the action of the sodium/potassium transporter protein adenosine triphosphatase, also called sodium/potassium pump or, Na^+K^+ATPase, which exchanges 3 molecules of Na^+ by 2 K^+ molecules. Thus, this exchange favors the formation of a reduced Na^+ concentration gradient and an intracellular electronegative gradient, a physiological scenario that facilitates the continuous entry of sodium into the cell and its reabsorption into the *vasa recta*, to the systemic circulation and the ECF [8].

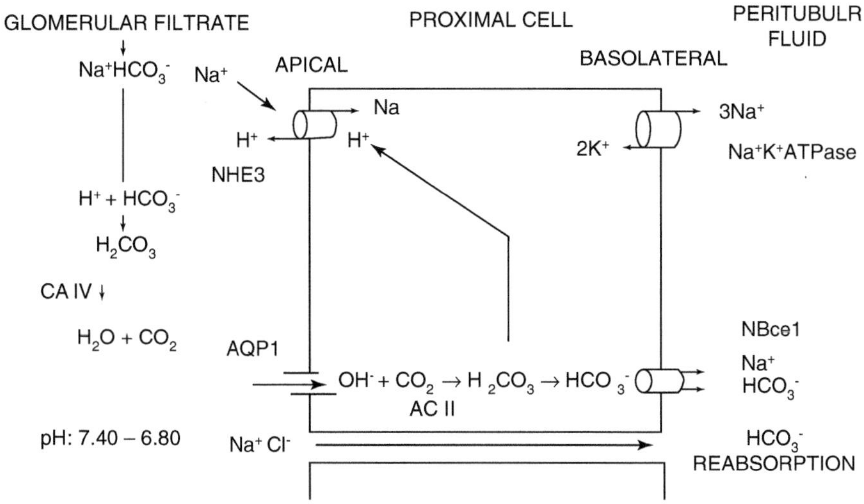

Fig. 2.1 Proximal tubule: Excretion of H^+ and reabsorption of Na^+HCO_3- initiates in the brush border cells of the proximal tubule. The Na^+HCO_3 molecule splits in the tubular lumen, allowing the Na^+ molecule to be exchanged for H^+ through the apical membrane, by the exchanger protein NHE3. Acetazolamide inhibits whereas angiotensin II (AG II) accelerates the expression of NHE3. The H^+ excreted in the tubular lumen binds to the HCO_3- molecule which remained from the sodium bicarbonate filtered previously in the glomerulus. The equilibrium reaction takes place in the tubular lumen, rendering carbonic acid (H_2CO_3) and $CO_2 + H_2O$ in the presence of the enzyme carbonic anhydrase IV (AC IV). CO_2 and H_2O are transported to the cytoplasm in the presence of aquaporins, mainly AQP 1. In the cytosol, the equilibrium reaction gets reversed, leading to reassemble H^++ HCO_3^-. H^+ is again excreted to the tubular lumen, while HCO_3^- is reabsorbed by the basolateral membrane, after binding Na^+, favored by the NBCe1 cotransporter. Na^+ molecules are also reabsorbed by the Na^+K^+ATPase protein, exchanging 3 Na^+ molecules for 2 K^+, facilitating intracellular electronegativity and Na^+ reabsorption from the lumen into the peritubular space. Chromosomal alterations of the NHE3 counter transporter, AC, and the NBCe1 cotransporter lead to the development of Type II primary proximal renal tubular acidosis

Hydrogen ions go in the opposite direction, being extracted from the cytosol of the proximal cells toward the proximal tubular lumen, in exchange for Na^+ molecules, by the NHE3 exchanger (Na^+/H^+ exchanger), as already mentioned. There, the hydrogen ions bind to HCO_3^- molecules that remained free in the tubular lumen to form carbonic acid (H_2CO_3). The equilibrium reaction starts this way within the tubular luminal fluid, a chemical reaction that is catalyzed in the presence of the enzyme carbonic anhydrase IV (AC IV), in the apical membrane of the brush border cells.

Carbonic acid dissociates in carbon dioxide (CO_2) and H_2O; both molecules penetrate the cell through the apical membrane favored by the action of H_2O transport proteins, which in the proximal tubule is mainly aquaporin 1 (AQP1), which also functions as transmembrane gas transporter. In the present situation, AQP1 transports CO_2 through the apical membrane, as well as water molecules, into the cytoplasm [9].

The reabsorption of H_2O molecules is catalyzed by the presence of various aquaporins, throughout the nephron. Once the H_2O and CO_2 molecules enter the cytoplasm, the equilibrium reaction is reversed, leading to the intracellular production of $H^+ + HCO_3^-$. Isoforms of carbonic anhydrase II and IV (AC II, AC IV) are important metalloenzymes in the regulation of acid-base metabolism, since they associate the respiratory component with the metabolic component, working simultaneously in both directions through the equilibrium reaction [10], as described below:

$$CO_2 + H_2O(AC) \leftrightarrow H_2CO_3 \leftrightarrow H^+ + HCO_3^-$$

This way, CO_2 is produced during the cellular metabolism, to be transported by the bloodstream and excreted by the lungs in the form of pCO_2. On the other hand, in the equilibrium reaction H^+ is eliminated by the kidneys, a process that leads to the production and reabsorption of bicarbonate. As this happens, carbonic anhydrase accelerates the equilibrium reaction hundreds of times per second, becoming an important mechanism of the buffer system in the EEC, as well as the renal regulation of the acid-base metabolism.

Although the CO_2 is not an acid, it behaves as such due to its participation in the equilibrium reaction in a clockwise direction, mainly in clinical situations of overproduction and accumulation of pCO_2 (respiratory acidosis). The increased production of CO_2 makes the equilibrium reaction run to the right, leading to the formation of HCO_3^- and H^+ ions. Bicarbonate molecules produced this way are used as a buffer, whereas the protons are excreted by the kidneys. The AC is essential in the reabsorption of bicarbonate and the excretion of hydrogen ions.

Once CO_2 and H_2O molecules enter the cytoplasm of the renal tubular cell through the apical membrane, the equilibrium reaction is reversed; the intracellular H_2O molecule dissociates into a hydrogen ion (H^+) and a hydroxyl group (OH^-), facilitated by the intracellular carbonic anhydrase II (AC II). The OH^- group binds to CO_2 to form bicarbonate. Once the $Na^+HCO_3^-$ molecules are reassembled in the cytoplasm, they are reabsorbed as such through the basolateral membrane, facilitated by the presence of the sodium/bicarbonate exchanger, Na^+ $3HCO_3^-$ (NBCe1), which transports 3 bicarbonate molecules, coupled by 1 sodium molecule [11] (Fig. 2.1). Besides, the excretion of H^+ is further facilitated by the presence of a vacuolar proton transporter protein in the apical membrane, the H^+ATPase or V-H^+ATPase (vacuolar), although to a lesser extent in the proximal tubule than in the collecting tubule, where this transporter exercises its priority action on the α-intercalated cells [12]. Alterations or mutations of the NHE3, NBCe1, and AC II transporter proteins give rise to the development of hereditary proximal RTA, as described in the corresponding chapter of this text.

Hydrogen ion excretion and the consequent bicarbonate reabsorption are closely linked to sodium reabsorption in the proximal tubule. Under physiological conditions, the amount of Na^+ reabsorbed, mainly as Na^+Cl^- and Na^+ HCO_3^- at this site of the nephron, is about 70% of the glomerular filtration rate. Therefore, the glomerular filtration rate is a determining factor in the reabsorption of bicarbonate, sodium, chloride, and other electrolytes. Under physiological conditions, 50% to 75% of the filtered Na^+ molecules are reabsorbed via the transcellular route; the remaining sodium by the paracellular route. Sodium reabsorption increases significantly during dehydration, hypovolemia, or shock [13].

In contrast, 80% to 90% of the $NaHCO_3^-$ filtered by the glomeruli is reabsorbed in the proximal tubule. Of this amount, 80% is reabsorbed by the transcellular route and the remaining 20% by the paracellular route, by passive diffusion. Although urinary acidification begins in the proximal tubule, it represents only a minimal quantity, since the urinary pH at the end of the proximal segment 3 (S3) is reduced barely to 6.8–6.7, from the filtered fluid at pH 7.40, at the time of leaving the glomerulus. In contrast, maximum urinary acidification is achieved in the distal medullary collecting tubules, with a maximal reduction of the pH to 4.5–4.0 [14].

The main objective of the physicochemical functions described in the proximal tubule is the recovery of the filtered bicarbonate by the glomeruli, which otherwise would be lost in the final urine. In the event, this occurs the pathologic entity is named proximal RTA (type II), which is due to a reduction of the proximal tubule bicarbonate reabsorption threshold; which is described at length in the corresponding chapter.

Ammonia Synthesis and Excretion in the Proximal Tubule

In the present section, the term ammonia is described as the buffer pair composed of ammonia (NH_3) and ammonium (NH_4^+) molecules (pK $\cong$ 9.15). Since most of the body fluids are stable with a pH of 7.40 (±0.05), most of the compound is in the form of ammonium.

The purpose of the buffer systems is to prevent or minimize sudden pH changes in the ECF. Thus, the buffer function $NH_3 + H^+ \rightarrow NH_4^+$ avoids the accumulation of H^+, which will be later excreted by the kidneys. Most of the substances that participate in some way in the physiology of the kidneys are provided by the systemic circulation, whereas ammonia is produced (ammonia-genesis) inside the kidneys, throughout the epithelial cells of the nephron, including some of the glomerular epithelial cells (Fig. 2.2). Nevertheless, most of the production is in the mitochondria of the brush border cells of the S1, S2, and S3 segments of the proximal tubule, mainly as NH_3. Ammonia formation originates from the amino acid glutamine metabolism. After several biochemical modifications, ammonia becomes transformed into α-ketoglutarate, rendering 3 bicarbonate and 2 ammonia molecules at the end of the process.

Systemic acidosis is a powerful stimulus to increase ammonia production in the proximal tubules [15]. NH_3 molecules are extracted from the cell at the apical membrane, mainly by the sodium/hydrogen exchanger (Na^+/H^+) (NHE3). The diuretic acetazolamide inhibits the action of carbonic anhydrase in the proximal tubule, favoring the development of metabolic acidosis. Besides, acetazolamide inhibits the NHE3 transporter protein; therefore, NH_4^+ excretion. The increased NHE3

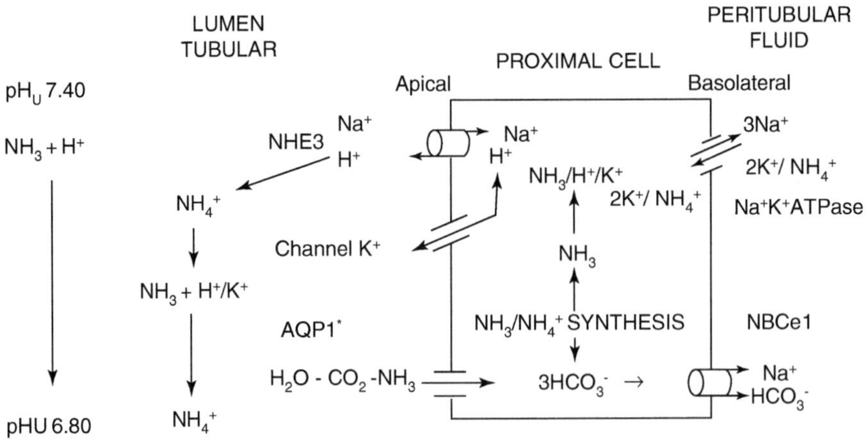

Fig. 2.2 Proximal tubule: Synthesis and secretion of ammonia. NH_3 molecules are exchanged for H^+ in the cells of the proximal tubule by NHE3 in the apical membrane, as well as for K^+ at the sites of various K^+ channels, such as KCNA10, TWIK 1, KCNQ1, and KCNE1, going from the cytosol into the tubular fluid, where it binds to H^+ to form NH_4^+. The bicarbonate formed in the cytoplasm during the equilibrium reaction is reabsorbed coupled to a Na^+ molecule, by the sodium/bicarbonate co-transporter, NBCel located in the basolateral membrane. This is the same site of exchange of K^+ for NH_4^+, which enters the cytosol from the peritubular fluid

expression and proximal tubular ammonium excretion seem to need the activation of the angiotensin II receptor (R-Ag II) [16].

It is worth mentioning that ammonia molecules may be exchanged for Na^+ or H^+ molecules, at the transport site channels where these cations are transported through the cell membrane of the renal tubular cells. This phenomenon occurs since the hydrodynamic radius of these cations is similar to those of ammonia. Also, there are cellular transmembrane transporter proteins that are specific for ammonia, primarily for NH_3, as will be described later. The largest amount of ammonia is extracted from the cell into the tubular lumen, where it binds to an H^+ molecule to form NH_4^+, although a small amount gets reabsorbed through the cell's basolateral membrane [17]. As mentioned before, the two ammonia molecules produced in the proximal tubule are excreted in the final urine, whereas the 3 bicarbonate molecules are restored to the ECF by the (NBCel) cotransporter, contributing further to the regulation of the acid-base metabolic process. NBCel mutations give rise to proximal renal tubular acidosis, type II [18].

New K^+ channels have recently been described in the brush border cells of the proximal tubules. They share potassium channel transport sites with other cations, mainly ammonia and, with less specificity, with sodium. They are the so-called "hyperpolarization-activated cation channels and cyclic nucleotides", also known as HCN or pacemaker channels, which comprise 4 homologous subunits, HCN1 to HCN4. The HCN1 and HCN3 channels are located in the apical membrane of the proximal tubular cells and transport NH_3 from the cytosol to the tubular lumen. There, they bind free H^+ ions to form ammonia, which in turn, are transported in the

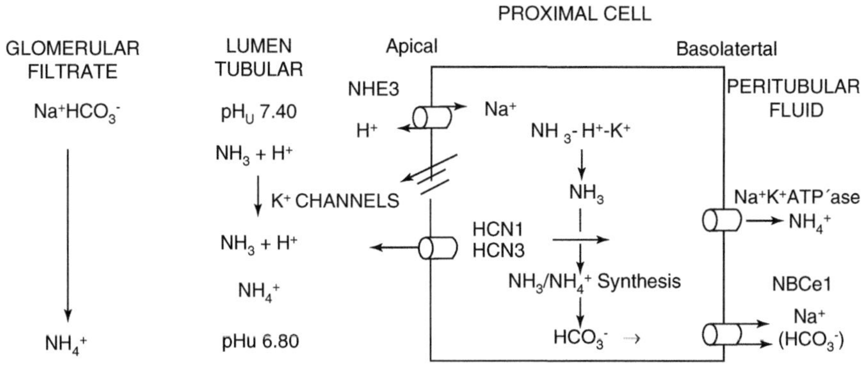

Fig. 2.3 Proximal tubules: Ammonia excretion. Cationic channels activated by hyperpolarization and cyclic nucleotides (HCN). HCNs (pacemaker channels) comprise 4 homologous subunits, HCN1 to HCN4. HCN1 and HCN3 are expressed in the apical membrane of the proximal tubule brush border cells, being their main function is the excretion of K^+ ions, which can be exchanged for other cations, such as NH_3, from the cytoplasm to the tubular lumen. At this site, it binds an H^+ ion to form NH_4^+, which descends via the proximal convoluted tubule into Henle's descending loop. In the basolateral membrane, NH_4^+ occupies the K^+ site of the Na^+K^+ATPase transporter protein

luminal fluid to the collecting tubules. In addition to proximal hydrogen excretion, HCNs favor the ammonia genesis process.

HCN2 is expressed in the basolateral membrane of the α-intercalated cells of the collecting tubules, captures NH_4^+ which is transported to the cytosol; from there on to the tubular lumen for its final excretion. Furthermore, pacemaker channels are present in the α-intercalated cells of the collecting tubule, as well as in the thick ascending limb of the loop of Henle, as will be described later [19] (Fig. 2.3).

The mechanisms of hydrogen ion reabsorption and ammonia excretion in the proximal tubule allow the recovery of bicarbonate from the glomerular filtrate and its reabsorption into the extracellular space. Furthermore, urinary acidification begins in the proximal tubule, albeit moderately, reducing the initial filtrate pH from 7.40 to ±6.80.

Hydrogen Excretion and Bicarbonate Reabsorption in the Loop of Henle

The descending limb of Henle's loop directs the glomerular filtrate from the proximal convoluted tubule to the renal medullary portion. While the fluid progresses downstream, NaCl is reabsorbed into the medullary interstitium, decreasing progressively its concentration inside the lumen. As the electrolyte concentration increases, NaCl has an important role in the countercurrent mechanism, a determining physiological function that participates in the maximum urinary concentration and dilution capacity. This mechanism also facilitates the concentration and recycling of ammonia in the medullary interstitium and, its final excretion in the urine, with an important effect on the systemic and renal regulation of acid-base metabolism [20].

The ascending limb of the loop of Henle reabsorbs approximately 15% of the bicarbonate filtered in the glomeruli and has unique physiological characteristics concerning the reabsorption of Na^+ and other electrolytes, as well as in the regulation of acid-base metabolism. This area of the nephron is impermeable to water.

Sodium reabsorption is dependent on the cotransporter Na^+ K^+ 2Cl- (NKCC2), which transports sodium and potassium, 1 molecule each, plus 2 molecules of chloride, through the apical membrane of the tubular lumen [21, 22] (Fig. 2.4). Cl^- molecules which enter the cytoplasm, leave the cell through the basolateral membrane by the K^+/Cl^- exchanger, whereas Na^+ is extracted from the cytosol towards the interstitium by the action of the basolateral exchanger Na^+K^+ATP'ase (sodium/potassium pump), which, as in the proximal tubule, exchanges 3 Na^+ molecules

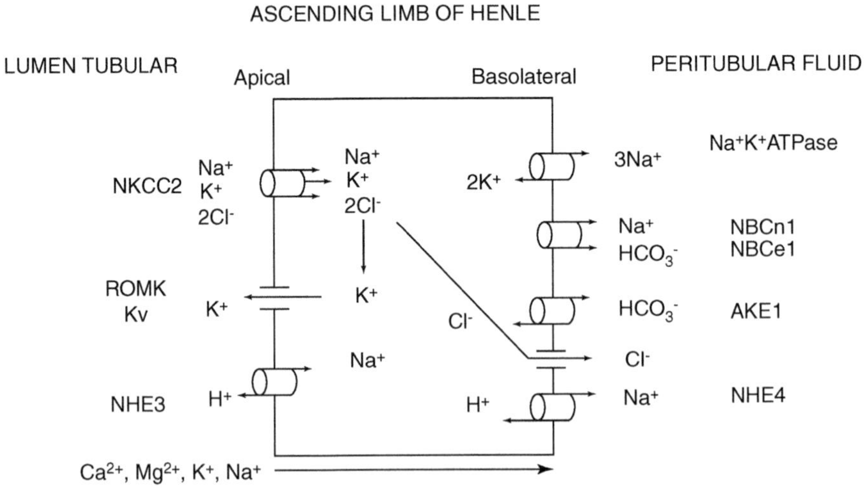

Fig. 2.4 Thick ascending limb of the loop of Henle (TALH): Hydrogen excretion and bicarbonate reabsorption. This important part of the nephron, characterized by being impermeable to water, is the dilution site of the urine in the tubular lumen; it's a relevant piece for the generation of a hypertonic interstitium and the development of the countercurrent mechanism. There is no aquaporins function in the apical membrane. Na^+, K^+, and Cl^- are reabsorbed from the tubular lumen, by the Na^+K^+ $2Cl^-$ cotransporter, which is inhibited by the use of loop diuretics. The K^+ accumulating in the cytosol is excreted to the apical membrane through the K^+ channels (ROMK). As in the proximal tubule, the NHE3 cotransporter also exchanges Na^+ for H^+ in the apical membrane. The Na^+ entering the cell through the NKCC2 cotransporter gets reabsorbed in the basolateral membrane in exchange for 2 K^+ molecules by the Na^+K^+ATP'ase anti-transporter. Sodium bicarbonate is reabsorbed in the basolateral membrane by the Na^+ HCO_3^- cotransporters, NBCe1 and NBCn1, as well as by exchange with Cl- by the anionic counter transporter AKE1. Furthermore, in the basolateral membrane, the Na^+ molecules are reabsorbed in exchange for H^+ by the NHE4 anti-transporter, which function is similar to its counterpart NHE3 in the apical membrane

extracted from the cytosol, for 2 K^+ molecules from the peritubular fluid. Both the entrance of potassium to the cell through the apical route ($Na^+K^+2Cl^-$) and the exit of chloride through the basolateral membrane (K^+Cl^-) generate a positive electric charge in the tubular lumen, facilitating the transcellular and paracellular reabsorption of Na^+. The concentration of cytoplasmic K^+ increases due to entry into the cell by the basolateral membrane (Na^+K^+ATP'ase), plus the K^+ entrance via the apical route ($Na^+K^+2Cl^-$). These molecules return to the tubular lumen through the K^+ channels localized in the apical membrane, called ROMK (Rat-Outer-Medullary K^+ Channel). Hence, the intracellular and luminal fluid recirculation of K^+ maintains the reabsorption cycle of Na^+, K^+, and Cl^- operating continuously in the ascending limb of Henle's loop [15, 22].

Another mechanism of Na^+ reabsorption in exchange for H^+ ions (NHE3) in the apical membrane, generating HCO_3^- molecules, which in turn become reabsorbed into the systemic circulation by the action of the Na^+/HCO_3^- cotransporter or exchanger (NBC1), located at the basolateral membrane [23].

Metabolism of Ammonia in the Loop of Henle

The ammonium from the proximal tubule is reabsorbed mainly in the form of ammonia (NH_3) progressively as the filtrate advances to the renal medullary portion in the path of the descending loop of Henle, a process that is facilitated by the countercurrent mechanism. NH_3 accumulates and is recycled in the medullary interstitial fluid, to finally be excreted in the collecting tubule. The purpose of increasing the concentration of NH_4^+ and NH_3 in the tubular lumen and the peritubular fluid is to facilitate the excretion of NH4$^+$ in the final urine through the collecting tubule.

Ammonia (NH_3/NH_4^+) does not cross the cell membrane since it is not fat-soluble; therefore, it requires transporter proteins to carry out the reabsorption and tubular excretion processes (Fig. 2.5). The main mechanism of apical transmembrane transport in the ascending limb of the loop of Henle is the Na $^+$ K^+ $2Cl^-$ exchanger (NKCC2), which can transport ammonia as a substitute for K^+ in the apical membrane. Therefore, it also participates in the regulation of acid-base metabolism [23, 24]. Luminal NH4$^+$ competes with K^+ for transport sites of the NKCC2 transporter protein. In the presence of hypokalemia or hyperkalemia, the concentration of K^+ in the tubular lumen is altered and, thus, altering the transport of NH4$^+$ at the same time [25, 26].

The thick ascending limb of Henle's loop is characterized by increasing ammonium reabsorption and the recycling of ammonia in the renal medulla (Fig. 2.5). The high concentration of ammonia in the medullary interstitium is due to the reabsorption of ammonia in the descending limb and, the parallel reabsorption in the thick ascending limb of Henle, acting simultaneously in the form of a short circuit. The high concentration of ammonia that is reached in this area facilitates excretion into

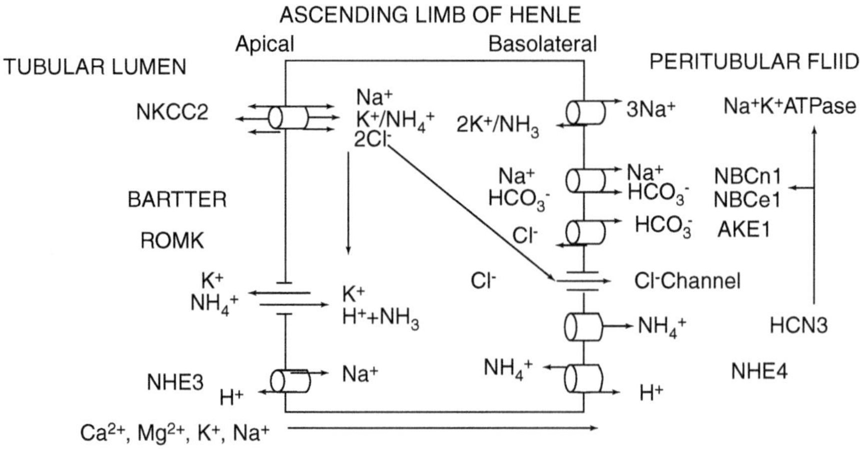

Fig. 2.5 Thick ascending limb of the loop of Henle (TALH): Reabsorption and excretion of ammonia. Renal metabolism in the loop of Henle shows particular characteristics since the reabsorption of NH_3 at the apical membrane predominates. NH_3 accumulates and recycles in the medullary peritubular space, to its subsequent absorption and excretion in the collecting tubule. Only a minor amount of NH_4 $^+$ (± 30%), remains in the tubular lumen, to continue its way to the distal tubule. In the apical membrane, NH_4^+ molecules may compete for the K^+ sites at the $Na^+K^+2Cl^-$ cotransporter (NKCC2). In the ROMK channels, NH_4^+ is absorbed and K^+ ions are removed from the cell into the lumen. Ammonia is also exchanged for H^+ ions in the anti-transporter NHE3 of the apical membrane. In the basolateral membrane, NH3 molecules are exchanged at the K^+ sites of the Na^+K^+ATPase transporter protein. Besides, the anti-transporter NH4 is expressed in the basolateral membrane, which exchanges Na^+ ions (which enter the cytosol), for H^+ ions, which are extracted into the peritubular fluid. NH_4^+ molecules are exchanged for H^+ ions, thereby increasing the reabsorption of ammonia in the TALH. HCN3 pacemaker channel facilitates the reabsorption of NH_4^+ and stimulates the NBCn1 cotransporter, as well as the Na^+K^+ATPase transporter in the basolateral membrane. At the moment, chromosomal alterations in the TALH that may lead to the development of ATR are unknown

the collecting tubule and excretion of NH_4^+ in the final urine. The anti-transporter Na^+/H^+ or Na^+/NH_4^+ (NHE4) is expressed in the basolateral membrane, the main action of which is to extract NH_4^+ from the cell to replace H^+. This mechanism facilitates increasing the concentration of NH_4^+ in the medullary peritubular fluid; the result of which involves the reabsorption of a significant amount of ammonia in Henle's thick ascending limb, thus, avoiding ammonia to proceed towards the distal tubule. Only 20 to 40% is transported to the distal tubule. Just a small amount of ammonia is reabsorbed in the distal tubule and about 10% to 15% goes downstream to the collecting tubule for its final excretion in the urine [27, 28].

Also, in the basolateral membrane are expressed the "cation channels activated by hyperpolarization and cyclic nucleotides" (HCN3), which participate in the reabsorption of NH_4^+ and the extraction of NH_3 from the cytosol to the interstitium where it accumulates during the countercurrent mechanism. These channels stimulate the sodium/bicarbonate exchanger (NBCn1, NBCe1) and the Na^+K^+ATPase protein, so, the presence of HCN3 is important in the regulation of acid-base metabolism [29].

Hydrogen and Ammonium Excretion in the Distal and Connector Tubules

Tubular sodium reabsorption continues in the distal convoluted tubule, as well as in the principal cells of the connecting tubule and cortical collecting duct. This area of the nephron is known as the "aldosterone-sensitive distal nephron" (ASDN), where sodium reabsorption is through the epithelial sodium channels (ENaC). The apical reabsorption of sodium molecules in the distal tubule is mainly in exchange for K^+ and to a lesser extent for hydrogen ions. This function is dependent on aldosterone, a hormone produced in the "zona glomerulosa" of the adrenal glands. Aldosterone stimulates the opening of the ENaC [30].

The scientific information available regarding the metabolism of ammonia in the distal tubule is scarce due to the difficulties in accessing this region of the kidney by micro-puncture studies. However, ammonia excretion in this tubular segment complies with some 10% to 15% of the total excretion of this buffer, under physiological conditions.

Hydrogen Excretion in the Collecting Tubule

Most hydrogen ions excretion and the consequent formation of "new bicarbonate" take place in the apical (luminal) membrane of the α-intercalated cells of the collecting tubule. In this area of the nephron, hydrogen ion excretion is independent of the reabsorption of sodium. The main excretory mechanism for H^+ ions depends on the hydrogen pump or adenosine tri-phosphatase (H^+ ATPase), which is also called vacuolar H^+ ATPase (V-H^+ ATPase) [30]. The H ATPase is made up of several subunits and it is energy-dependent. The B1 subunit is similar to the basolateral H^+ ATPase of the proximal tubule, while the B2 subunit performs its function mainly in the collecting duct of the kidney. α-intercalated cells increase the production of V-H^+ ATPase in response to several factors, such as the reduction of intracellular pH; the increase in the organic production of hydrogen ions and the presence of metabolic acidosis. This situation also occurs as a renal tubular metabolic compensation mechanism in the presence of secondary respiratory acidosis, with pCO_2 retention [31–34] (Fig. 2.6).

There is another mechanism of excretion of hydrogen through the apical membrane in the collecting tubules, which is the H^+ K^+ ATPase transporter protein, which exchanges an H^+ molecule extracted from the cytoplasm, in exchange for a K^+ molecule from the tubular lumen. This exchange is electroneutral, so it does not affect its function in the presence of transmembrane voltage changes. Two isoforms are expressed in the digestive system, gastric H^+K^+ ATPase, which is involved in the production of H^+Cl^- in the gastric mucosa and, colonic H^+K^+ ATPase. These isoforms are also expressed in the kidney. The presence of metabolic acidosis increases the production of H^+K^+ATPase. It is also stimulated in the presence of hypokalemia.

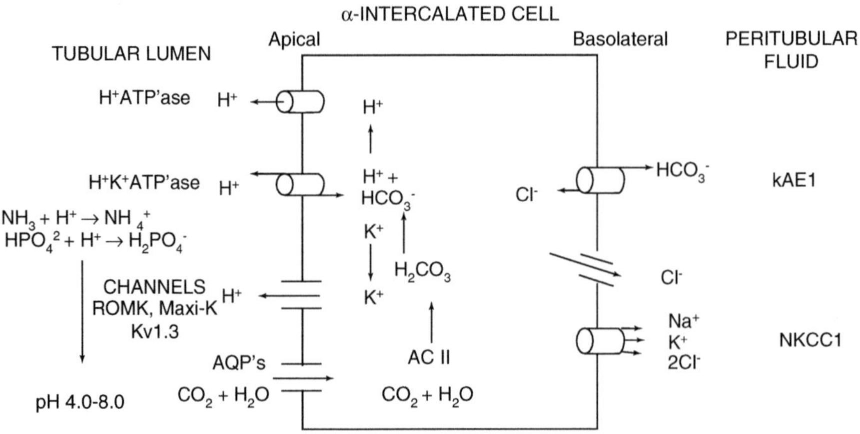

Fig. 2.6 Connecting and collecting tubules, α-intercalated cell: Hydrogen excretion and bicarbonate reabsorption. This is an important part of the nephron in hydrogen excretion, which in turn is accompanied by bicarbonate molecule formation. This "new bicarbonate" is reabsorbed into the peritubular fluid and the extracellular fluid. The main function of "new bicarbonate" is to correct systemic acidosis. In this area, the excretion of H^+ ions is independent of the reabsorption of Na^+. In the apical membrane, the excretion of H^+ depends mainly on the transporter proteins H^+ ATPase (V H^+ ATPase) or hydrogen bomb and H^+K^+ATPase, or potassium/hydrogen pump. Both transporter proteins excrete H^+ into the tubular lumen; H^+K^+ATPase in exchange for K^+ ions. H^+ ions excreted in the tubular lumen bind phosphates to form phosphoric acid ($HPO_4^2 + H^+ \rightarrow H_2PO_4^-$) and sulfates to form sulfuric acid ($HSO_4^2 + H^+ \rightarrow H_2SO_4^-$), or titratable acid, to form ammonium ($NH_3 + H^+ \rightarrow NH_4^+$). K^+ entering the cell is extracted through the K^+ channels (ROMK, Maxi-K, Kv1.3) into the tubular lumen. In the apical membrane, there is almost no AC IV; thus, CO_2 and H_2O molecules form slowly in the tubular space. However, intracellular AC II is abundant and sodium bicarbonate is produced and reabsorbed through the basolateral membrane by kAE1, which transports Cl^- to the cytosol and HCO_3^- to the peritubular medullary fluid. Cl^- ions are reabsorbed by Cl^- channels, together with Na^+ and K^+ by the $Na^+K^+2Cl^-$ cotransporter, or NKCC1, in the basolateral membrane. NKCC1 is the counterpart of NKCC2, the latter expressed in the apical membrane of TALH. Chromosomal mutations of the H^+ATPase, AC II, and the anti-transporter kAE1 are the etiology of primary distal ATR, type I

H^+K^+ATPase exchanges K^+ for H^+ and can exchange Na^+ molecules for H^+; acting this way as a Na^+K^+ ATPase. It can also exchange NH_4^+ for K^+ to excrete it. The reduction in blood K^+ concentration as well as the presence of metabolic acidosis stimulate the secretion of H^+K^+ ATPase in the collecting tubule [35, 36].

The reabsorption of Na^+ through the basolateral membrane is facilitated by the presence of the Na^+K^+ ATPase protein, as well as by the NKCC1 exchanger, which is the counterpart to the NKCC2, whose function is exerted in the apical membrane of the thick ascending limb of Henle. Likewise, its counterpart NKCC1 carries one Na^+, one K^+, and two Cl^- molecules; but the molecular transportation takes place in the opposite direction, that is, from the α-intercalated cell cytoplasm to the fluid of the peritubular space.

Intracellular carbonic anhydrase (AC II) plays an important role as a source of intracellular H^+ production (through the equilibrium reaction) which, in turn, is excreted by the transporter proteins V-H^+ ATPase and H^+K^+ATPase. In contrast, extracellular AC IV is almost non-existent in the collecting tubule [37]. The new HCO_3- produced in the α-intercalated cell is reabsorbed at the basolateral membrane by the presence of the anionic anti-transporter kAE1, which regulates the tight junction through the Claudin-4 protein [38].

Contrary to what happens in the presence of acidosis, when the intracellular or systemic pH increases, or in the presence of a fully developed clinical metabolic alkalosis, H^+K^+ ATP'ase translates the site of action toward the basolateral membrane at the β-intercalated cells, increasing the amount of bicarbonate excretion and conserving hydrogen ions that return to ECF, in the process of correcting or compensating the alkalosis. The H^+ ATP'ase (V-H^+ ATP'ase) transporter protein, which generally functions in the luminal membrane of the α-intercalated cells to excrete H^+ ions, can also transfer its function to β-intercalated cells to excrete bicarbonate during an episode of systemic alkalosis, thus demonstrating the functionality of these transporter proteins [39, 40].

Mutations of AC II, V-H^+ ATPase and anion exchanger kAE1 give rise to the development of distal tubular acidosis (Type I). The chromosomal mutations leading to the development of renal tubular acidosis are described in detail in the corresponding chapter.

H^+ transporter molecules, mostly V-H^+ATP'ase, excrete intracellular H^+ into the tubular lumen, where hydrogen ions bind to phosphate to form phosphoric acid ($HPO_4^{-2}/H_2PO_4^-$) and sulfates to form sulfuric acid ($HSO_4^{-2}/H_2SO_4^-$), which are excreted as urinary buffers in the form of titratable acid [19]. Also, hydrogen ions bind ammonia (NH_3) to form ammonium (NH_4^+). Under physiological conditions, approximately half the buffering is as titratable acid and the rest as ammonia/ammonium. However, when systemic acidosis develops, most of the buffering relies on ammonia/ammonium [41].

Excretion of Ammonia in the Collecting Tubule

About 80% ammonia excretion is in the α-intercalated cells of the collecting tubule, making this region of the nephron the most important site of regulation of the metabolic component of systemic acid-base balance [42].

Various transporter proteins participate in the collecting tubule to carry out the process of urinary acidification, consisting mainly of capturing NH_3 from the medullary interstitium, introducing it into the cytosol of the α-intercalated cells, to its final urinary excretion as NH_4^+. Therefore, the process of reabsorption of ammonia is, as already mentioned, in the ascending limb of the loop of Henle, whereas the excretion is carried out in the opposite direction toward the tubular lumen in the α-intercalated cell of the collecting tubule, completing the recycling process of NH_3/NH_4^+, as part of the countercurrent mechanism [43, 44].

Transmembrane transport proteins, such as V-H^+ ATPase and H^+K^+ATPase, are expressed in the apical membrane of the α-intercalated cells of the collecting tubule.

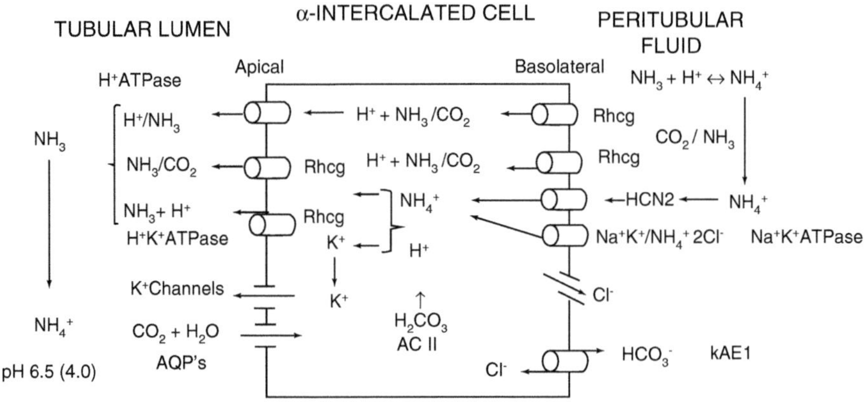

Fig. 2.7 Connecting and collecting tubules, α.intercalated cell: Ammonium excretion. In the presence of systemic acidosis, the highest excretion of H^+, up to 80%, occurs as ammonia, in the α-intercalated cell of the collecting tubules. In the apical membrane, the ammonia (NH_3) molecules compete for the H^+ sites at the H^+ATPase transporter, and mainly for the K^+ sites at the H^+K^+ ATPase transporter. NH_3 is excreted in the tubular lumen, where it binds to H^+ to form NH_4^+. The Rhesus glycoproteins (Rh) are expressed in the α-intercalated cell as the subunits Rhbg and Rhcg, which are gas transport proteins, including carbon dioxide, ammonia, and nitric oxide in various organs, including the kidney. Rhcg glycoprotein, which participates in NH_3 excretion, is expressed in the apical membrane. In the basolateral membrane, both Rh glycoproteins facilitate the capture of NH_4^+ molecules from the peritubular fluid, into the cytosol of the α-intercalated cell. Furthermore, NH_4^+ competes for the K^+ sites in the NKCC1 transporter ($Na^+K^+2Cl^-$) in the basolateral membrane. Hyperpolarization-activated cation channels and cyclic nucleotides (pacemaker channels) are expressed in the α-intercalated cell and, in the principal cells of the collecting tubules. The HCN2 isoform captures NH_4^+ from the peritubular fluid and releases it into the cytosol, to be excreted through the apical membrane into the final urine

At this site, NH_4^+ may compete for the binding sites of the membrane for H^+ and K^+, to be excreted as a buffer in the final urine [45, 46] (Fig. 2.7).

Within the most inner area of the renal medulla, the apical membranes of the α-intercalated cells are devoided of extracellular carbonic anhydrase IV (AC IV) [47]. Nonetheless, intracellular α-intercalated cells are very abundant in anhydrase II carbonic acid enzyme, which participates in the equilibrium reaction in the cytosol, resulting in the formation of bicarbonate and hydrogen ions. These protons allow the urinary acidification process to keep going, by H^+ leaving the α-intercalated cell cytosol towards the tubular lumen through the action of V-H^+ATPase and the H^+K^+ ATP'ase in the apical membrane [48]. On the other hand, HCO_3^- gets reabsorbed from the cytosol into the peritubular fluid through the basolateral membrane, in the presence of the kAE1 anion exchanger, which exchanges HCO_3^- for Cl^- [49].

NH_4^+ is exchanged for Na^+ or K^+ molecules at the K^+ sites of the Na^+K^+ATPase and NKCC1 transporters, to be transported from the peritubular fluid to the cytosol and then to the tubular lumen. Therefore, it participates in hydrogen ion excretion, although to a lesser extent than the other mechanisms already mentioned [50].

Hyperpolarization-activated cation channels and cyclic nucleotides (HCN) are also expressed in the α-intercalated cells in different tissues in rats and other mammals, where pacemaker HCN activity is regulated. In studies conducted in rats, it is suggested that HCN participates in the activation of the Na^+K^+ATPase protein and the Na^+/HCO_3^- (NBCn1) cotransporter, thus, participating in the regulation of acid-base metabolism. HCN2 is expressed in the α-intercalated cells of the collecting tubule, whose function is to capture NH_4^+ from the peritubular fluid to its transportation and release in the cytosol. Further excretion to the luminal fluid is carried out by Na^+K^+ATPase and V-H^+ATPase [51].

Contrary to the previously held concept that water and gases, like CO_2, cross cell membranes by passive diffusion through the bilipid membranes. However, water and gas channels have been detected in some cell membranes. Two families of H_2O and CO_2 transmembrane transporter proteins are known to date, aquaporins (AQPs) and Rhesus (Rh) glycoproteins. The first known function of AQPs was the transmembrane transport of H_2O, and subsequently, transport of CO_2 was known. This information led to an important change in the understanding of acid-base metabolism, since cellular transport of CO_2 and H_2O requires the presence of AQPs, both systemically and in the epithelial cells of the renal tubules [52, 53]. Other investigations reported that AQP 1 possesses the ability to transport nitric oxide (NO) through certain cell membranes, mainly in vascular endothelial cells, demonstrating the importance of this protein on the regulation of blood pressure [54].

Together with other ammonium transporter proteins, such as H^+ATPase and H^+K^+ATPase, Rhesus glycoproteins represent the main site of excretion of ammonia. The ammonia/ammonium buffer system is the main site for proton binding and excretion; its contribution is of the greatest importance in the regulation of acid-base metabolism [55]. Rhesus glycoproteins are expressed in several tissues of plants, animals and numerous microorganisms. These glycoproteins are gas transporters, mainly CO_2 and NH_3 [56–58].

Rhesus glycoproteins (Rhgc, Rhbg) capture and transport CO_2 and NH_4 from the peritubular fluid (hypertonic, with a high concentration of ammonia) to the cytosol. This mechanism ensues at the basolateral membrane of the α-intercalated cells of the collecting tubule. On the other hand, Rhgc, but not Rhbg, is expressed at the apical membrane, and participates in the α-intercalated cells of the collecting tubule excreting NH_3 and CO_2 [59] (Fig. 2.7).

The Physiological Impact of Urinary Buffers in the Excretion of Hydrogen

A buffering substance contains a weak acid and a weak base, with their respective salts; can minimize sudden changes in pH in a solution.

A normal subject, under physiologic normal status, needs to excrete 80 to 100 mEq of hydrogen ions, daily. It would be necessary to drop the urine pH to 1.5, to excrete such an amount of non-volatile acids. On the contrary, to excrete an alkaline charge, it is required to increase the urinary pH to 8.0. This situation is not feasible, since the renal capacity to acidify and alkalinize the urine, falls within a 4.0 to 8.0 pH range, which corresponds to an $[H^+]$ of 1/0.0001 (10^{-4}) and 1/0.00000001 (10^{-8}).

Therefore, the kidneys utilize buffers to excrete the non-volatile H^+ ions. The renal excretion of excess hydrogen (H^+) is achieved by titratable acid (TA) and ammonia excretion. These buffers are of minimal physiological importance at the systemic level, but in the urine, their role is most important to excrete protons. The largest amount of systemic hydrogen ions are derived from the intermediate metabolism of amino acids. The concentration of free H^+ $[H^+]$ in the ECF is 0.0000000398 (nm/l). The logarithmic expression of this value is 3.98×10^{-8}, corresponding to a pH of 7.40 (±0.05).

Most of the ammonia is produced mainly in the proximal tubule and is excreted as ammonium molecules in the urine. The presence of buffer systems in the urine leads to a reduction of the amount of free H^+, maintaining the urinary pH stable at 6.0–6.5, under physiological conditions. The production of urinary buffers, mostly ammonia, is increased in the presence of metabolic acidosis, which occurs in the α-intercalated cells of the connecting and collecting tubules. On the contrary, when bicarbonate accumulates in the ECF (metabolic alkalosis), the excess is excreted in the β-intercalated cells. From this, it can be deduced that the urinary pH is not an indicator of the quantity of excreted buffers, but rather of the urinary quantity of free hydrogens (H^+), in the case of systemic acidosis, or of hydroxyls (OH-), which are transformed in HCO_3-, in the case of systemic metabolic alkalosis.

Once the hydrogen ions that are extracted from the α-interspersed cells into the lumen of the connecting and collecting tubules, they undergo the buffering process in the form of titratable acid (phosphoric and sulfuric acids) and ammonium (NH_4^+), which are excreted by the urine. Only a small amount of free hydrogen ions remain in the urine, determining the urinary pH within the physiological range of 6.0–6.5 [60].

The ammonia/ammonium buffer pair, which is been produced in the brush border of the proximal tubular cells, is the main mechanism of regulation of the acid-base metabolism since it excretes from 50% to 70% of the hydrogen produced in the body. This amount increases to 80% or 90% when the systemic production of H^+ rises, even slightly; when the renal intracellular pH is reduced or in the presence of a fully developed systemic acidosis, either of metabolic or respiratory origin (in this last instance as a compensatory mechanism). The renal response to increasing the urinary excretion of H^+ is by augmenting the expression of the cotransporters NBCn1 and NBC3 [60].

As previously mentioned, the main function of the proximal tubule concerning the regulation of acid-base metabolism is the recovery of bicarbonate filtered by the glomerulus, while the distal tubule has as a priority the formation of new bicarbonate, which happens as a consequence of the excretion of hydrogen ions bound to the buffer systems, mainly titratable acid and excretion of ammonia [61].

The ammonia/ammonium buffer system is formed by weak acid and its base, with a dissociation constant (pK) of ~9.15. The lower this value, the greater the amount of the buffer solution that is in the form of acid, NH_4^+, according to the following reaction:

$$NH_4^+ \rightarrow NH_3 + H^+$$

Therefore, in urine with a physiological pH of 6.0 to 7.0, the ammonium (acid form) excreted from the cell to the tubular lumen would be trapped until its final expulsion in the urine. As formerly described, this NH_4^+ "entrapment theory" is correct, but incomplete, due to the existence of NH_3/NH_4^+ transporter molecular proteins expressed throughout the nephron [61].

References

1. Chan JCM. Nutrition and acid-base metabolism. Fed Proc. 1981;40:2423–8.
2. Rodriguez-Soriano J. Renal tubular acidosis: the clinical entity. J Am Soc Nephrol. 2002;13:2160–70.
3. Goyal S, Vanden Heuvel G, Aronson PS. Renal expression of novel Na+/H+ exchanger isoform NHE8. Am J Physiol Renal Physiol. 2003;284(3):F467–73. Epub 2002 Oct 29.
4. Biemesderfer D, Pizzonia J, Abu-Alfa A, Exner M, Reilly R, Igarashi P, Aronson PS. NHE3: a Na+/H+ exchanger isoform of renal brush border. Am J Phys. 1993;265(5 Pt 2):F736–42.
5. Halperin ML, Kamel KS, Goldstein MB. Polyuria. In: Halperin ML, Kamel KS, Goldstein MB, editors. Fluid, electrolyte, and acid-base physiology. 4th ed. Philadelphia: Saunders Elsevier; 2010. p. 403–22.
6. Burckhardt G, DiSole F, Helmle-Kolb C. The Na^+/H^+ exchanger gene family. J Nephrol. 2002;15(Suppl 5):S3–S21.
7. Wang T, Hropor M, Aronson PS, Giebisch G. Role of NHE isoforms in mediating bicarbonate reabsorption along the nephron. Am J Phys. 2001;281:F1120–8.
8. Jorgensen PL. Structure, function and, regulation of Na+, K+ATPase in the kidney. Kidney Int. 1986;29:10–20.
9. Nielsen S, Agre P. The aquaporin family of water channels. Kidney Int. 1995;48(4):1057–106.
10. Silverman DN, Lindskoo S. The catalytic mechanism of carbonic anhydrase: implications of a rate-limiting protolysis of water. A Chem Res. 1988;21(1):30–6.
11. Soleimani M. Na^+HCO_3 cotransporter (NBC): expression and regulation in the kidney. J Nephrol. 2002;15(Suppl 5):S32–40.
12. Nakhoul NL, Hamm LL. Vacuolar H+ATPase in the kidney. J Nephrol. 2002;12(Suppl 5):S22–31.
13. Trachtman H. Sodium metabolism. In: Avner ED, Harmon WE, Niaudet P, editors. Pediatric nephrology. 5th ed. Philadelphia: Lippincott Williams & Wilkins; 2004. p. 125–45.
14. Dubose TD Jr, Cogan MG, Rector FC. Acid-base disorder. In: Brenner BM, Rector FC, editors. Brenner and Rector's the kidney. 5th ed. Philadelphia: WB Saunders; 1996. p. 929–98.
15. Hebert SC, Gamba G, Kaplan M. The electroneutral Na^+ -(K^+)-Cl cotransport family. Kidney Int. 1996;49:1638–41.
16. Nagami GT. Luminal secretion of ammonia in the mouse proximal tubule perfused in vitro. J Clin Invest. 1988;81:159–64.
17. Weiner ID, Verlander JW. Renal ammonia metabolism and transport. Compr Physiol. 2013;3(1):201–20. https://doi.org/10.1002/cphy.c120010.

18. Li HC, Szigligeti P, Worrell RT, Matthews JB, Conforti L, Soleimani M. Missense mutations in Na+:HCO3- cotransporter NBC1 show abnormal trafficking in polarized kidney cells: a basis of proximal renal tubular acidosis. Am J Physiol Renal Physiol. 2005;289(1):F61–71.
19. López-González Z, Cosete Ayala-Aguilera C, Martinez-Morales F, Galicia-Cruz O, Salvador-Hernández C, Pedraza-Chaverri J, Medeiros M, Hernández AM, Escobar L. Immunolocalization of hyperpolarization-activated cationic HCN1 and HCN3 channels in the rat nephron: regulation of HCN3 by potassium diets. Histochem Cell Biol. 2015;144(4) https://doi.org/10.1007/s00418-015-1375-6.
20. Trachtman H. Sodium and water. En: Avner ED, Harmon WE, Niaudet P. eds., Pediatric nephrology, 5th ed., Lippincott Williams & Wilkins, Philadelphia, 2004: 125–145.
21. Chan JCM, Mak RHK. Acid-base homeostasis. En: Avner ED, Harmon WE, Niaudet P. eds., Pediatric nephrology, 5th ed., Lippincott Williams & Wilkins, Philadelphia, 2004:189–208.
22. Weinstein AM, Krahn TA. A mathematical model of rat ascending Henle limb. II Epithelial function. Am J Physiol Renal Physiol. 2010;298:F525–42.
23. Amemiya M, Loffing J, Lotscher M, Kaissling B, Alpern RJ, Moe OW. Expression of NHE-3 in the apical membrane of rat renal proximal tubule and thick ascending limb. Kidney Int. 1996;48:1206–15.
24. Kikeri D, Sun A, Zeidel ML, Hebert SC. Cell membranes impermeable to NH3. Nature. 1989;339:478–80.
25. Attmane-Elakeb A, Amlal H, Bichara M. Ammonium carriers in medullary thick ascending limb. Am J Physiol Renal Physiol. 2001;280:F1–9.
26. DuBose TD, Good DW. Chronic hyperkalemia impairs ammonium transport and accumulation in the inner medulla of the rat. J Clin Invest. 1992;90:1443–9.
27. Good DW. Effects of potassium on ammonia transport by medullary thick ascending limb of the rat. J Clin Invest. 1987;80:1358–65.
28. Good DW. Active absorption of NH4_ by rat medullary thick ascending limb: inhibition by potassium. Am J Physiol Renal Fluid Electrolyte Physiol. 1988;255:F78–87.
29. Good DW, Knepper MA, Burg MA. Ammonia and bicarbonate transport by thick ascending limb of rat kidney. Am J Phys. 1984;247:F35–44.
30. Quinn S, Harvey BJ, Thomas W. Rapid aldosterone actions on epithelial sodium channel trafficking and cell proliferation. Steroids. 2014;81:43–8. https://doi.org/10.1016/j.steroids.2013.11.005. Epub 2013 Nov 20.
31. Halperin ML, Kamel KS, Goldstein MB: Principles of acid-base physiology. En Halperin ML, Kamel KS, Goldstein MB (eds): Fluid, electrolyte, and acid-base physiology 4th ed. Saunders Elsevier, Philadelphia, 2010:3–28.
32. Doucet A, Horisberger J. Renal ion-translocating ATPases. The P-type family. In: Seldin D, Giebisch G, editors. The kidney physiology and pathophysiology. Philadelphia: Lippincott Williams & Wilkins; 2000. p. 140–70.
33. Gluck S. Nelson r: the role of the V-ATPase in renal epithelial H+ transport. J Exp Biol. 1992;172:205–18.
34. Cavingston TL, Campbell WG, Wingo CS, Cainn BD. Molecular identification of the renal H^+K^+ -ATPases. Semin Nephrol. 1999;19:431–7.
35. Silver RB, Mennit PA, Satlin LM: Stimulation of H^+, K^+ATPase in intercalated cells of cortical collecting duct with chronic metabolic acidosis. Am J Physiol. 1996;270:F539–47. The kidney anion exchanger 1 affects tight junction properties via claudin-4.
36. Garg LC. Respective roles of H-ATPase and H-K-ATPase in ion transport in the kidney. J Am Soc Nephrol. 1991;2(5):949–60.
37. Wall SM, Fischer MP. Contribution of the Na_-K_-2Cl_ cotransporter (NKCC1) to transepithelial transport of H_, NH4_, K_, and Na_ in rat outer medullary collecting duct. J Am Soc Nephrol. 2002;13:827–35.
38. Lashhab R, Rumley AC, Arutyunov D, Rizvi M, You C, Dimke H, Touret N, Zimmermann R, Jung M, Chen XZ, Alexander T, Cordat E. The kidney anion exchanger 1 affects tight junction properties via claudin-4. Sci Rep. 2019;9:Article number: 3099.

39. Codina J, Dubose TD Jr. Molecular regulation and physiology of the HKATPases in the kidney. Semin Nephrol. 2006;26:345–51.
40. Gumz ML, Lynch IJ, Greenlee MM, Cain BD, Wingo CS. The renal-ATPases: physiology, regulation, structure. Am J Physiol Renal Physiol. 2010;298:F12–21.
41. McCance RA, von Finck MA. The titratable acidity, pH, ammonia and phosphates in the urines of very young infants. Arch Dis Child. 1947;22(112):200–9.
42. Koeppen BM, Steinmetz PR. Basic mechanisms of urinary acidification. Med Clin North Am. 1983;67(4):753–70.
43. Knepper MA. NH4 transport in the kidney. Kidney Int. 1991;40:S95–S102.
44. Knepper MA, Good DW, Burg MB. Mechanism of ammonia secretion by cortical collecting ducts of rabbits. Am J Physiol Renal Fluid Electrolyte Physiol. 1984;247:F729–38.
45. Kurtz I, Balaban RS. Ammonium as a substrate for Na_-K_-ATPase in rabbit proximal tubules. Am J Physiol Renal Fluid Electrolyte Physiol. 1986;250:F497–502.
46. Attmane-Elakeb A, Sibella V, Vernimmen C, Belenfant X, Hebert SC, Bichara M. Regulation by glucocorticoids of expression and activity of rBSC1, the Na_-K_ (NH4_)-2Cl_ cotransporter of medullary thick ascending limb. J Biol Chem. 2000;275:33548–53.
47. Brown D, Zhu XL, Sly WS. Localization of membrane-associated carbonic anhydrase type IV in kidney epithelial cells. Proc Natl Acad Sci U S A. 1990;87(19):7457–61.
48. Dobyan DC, Bulger RE. Renal carbonic anhydrase. Am J Phys. 1982;243(4):F311–24.
49. Vichot AA, Zsengellér ZK, Shmukler BE, Adams ND, Dahl NK, Alper SL. Loss of kAE1 expression in collecting ducts of end-stage kidneys from a family with SLC4A1 G609R-associated distal renal tubular acidosis. Clin Kidney J. 2017;10(1):135–40. https://doi.org/10.1093/ckj/sfw074. Epub 2016 Aug 31.
50. Wall SM, Fischer MP. Contribution of the Na(+)-K(+)-2Cl(−) cotransporter (NKCC1) to transepithelial transport of H(+), NH(4)(+), K(+), and Na(+) in rat outer medullary collecting duct. Am Soc Nephrol. 2002;13(4):827–35.
51. Carrisoza-Gaytan R, Rangel C, Salvador C, Saldaña-Meyer R, Escalona C, Satlin LM, Liu W, Zavilowitz B, Joyce Trujillo J, Bobadilla NA, Escobar LI. The hyperpolarization-activated cyclic nucleotide-gated HCN2 channel transports ammonium in the distal nephron. Kidney Int. 2011;80:832–40. https://doi.org/10.1038/ki.2011.230.
52. Itel F, Al-Samir S, Öberg F, Chami M, Kumar M, Supuran CT, Deen PM, Meier W, Hedfalk K, Gros G, Endeward V. CO2 permeability of cell membranes is regulated by membrane cholesterol and protein gas channels. FASEB J. 2012;26(12):5182–91. https://doi.org/10.1096/fj.12-209916. Epub 2012 Sep 10.
53. Boron WF, Cooper GJ. Effect of DIDS on the CO2 permeability of the water channel AQP1. FASEB J. 1998;12:A374.
54. Herrera M, Hong NJ, Garvin JL. Aquaporin-1 transports NO across cell membranes. Hypertension. 2006;2006(48):157–64.
55. Silver RB, Mennit PA, Satlin LM. Stimulation of H^+, K^+ ATPase in intercalated cells of cortical collecting duct with chronic metabolic acidosis. Am J Physiol. 1996;270:F539–47.
56. Endeward V, Cartron JP, Ripoche P, Gros G. RhAG protein of the Rhesus complex is a CO2 channel in the human red cell membrane. FASEB J. 2008;22:64–73.
57. Weiner ID, Hamm LL. Molecular mechanisms of renal ammonia transport. Annu Rev Physiol. 2007;69:317–40.
58. Muñoz-Arizpe R, Escobar L, Medeiros M. Acidosis tubular renal en niños: conceptos actuales de diagnóstico y tratamiento. Bol Med Hosp Infant Mex. 2013;70(3):178–94.
59. Eladari D, Cheval L, Quentin F, Bertrand O, Mouro I, Chérif-Zahar B, Cartron JP, Paillard M, Doucet A, Chambrey R. Expression of RhCG, a new putative NH3/NH+4 transporter, along the rat nephron. J Am Soc Nephrol. 2002;13:1999–2008.
60. Kwon TH, Fulton C, Wang W, Kurtz I, Frøkiær J, Aalkjaer C, Nielsen S. Chronic metabolic acidosis upregulates rat kidney Na-HCO cotransporters NBCn1 and NBC3 but not NBC1. Am J Physiol Renal Physiol. 2002;282:F341–51.
61. Alpern RJ, Rector FC. Renal acidification mechanisms. In: Brenner BM, editor. Brenner & Rector's, the kidney. 5th ed. Philadelphia: WB Saunders Co.; 1996. p. 408–71.

Chapter 3
Physiology of Renal Potassium Handling

Adrián Rafael Murillo-de-Ozores, Gerardo Gamba, and María Castañeda-Bueno

Introduction

K^+ is the most abundant cation in intracellular fluid with a concentration of approximately 140 mmol/L, while in the extracellular fluid (ECF) the physiological concentration of K^+ ranges between 3.5 and 5.0 mmol/L. This concentration gradient allows the establishment of the electrical potential of plasma membranes of all the cells of the organism, which plays an especially important role in excitable cells, such as in skeletal or cardiac muscle cells, smooth muscle cells, and neurons. Therefore, alterations in the extracellular K^+ concentration ($[K^+]_{ECF}$) can cause, for example, serious alterations in the function of skeletal or smooth muscle and the heart [1, 2].

Potassium Balance

Daily K^+ intake (±54 mmol/day) is similar to the total amount of K^+ in the extracellular fluid (±60 mmol). Therefore, different mechanisms are responsible for preventing sudden changes in the $[K^+]_{ECF}$ in the postprandial period.

The original version of the chapter has been revised. A correction to this chapter can be found at https://doi.org/10.1007/978-3-030-91940-5_12

A. R. Murillo-de-Ozores · G. Gamba · M. Castañeda-Bueno (✉)
Departamento de Nefrología y Metabolismo Mineral, Instituto Nacional de Ciencias Médicas y Nutrición Salvador Zubirán, Mexico City, Mexico
e-mail: maria.castanedab@incmnsz.mx

R. Muñoz (ed.), *Renal Tubular Acidosis in Children*,
https://doi.org/10.1007/978-3-030-91940-5_3

After a K^+ intake, translocation of K^+ into cells, mainly skeletal muscle cells, prevents a sudden increase in $[K^+]_{ECF}$. Different hormonal factors, such as insulin, epinephrine, and aldosterone, are responsible for this process. These three hormones have an activating effect on Na^+/K^+ ATPase, which mediates the transport of K^+ from the extracellular to the intracellular fluid. Insulin deficiency, a dysfunctional renin-angiotensin-aldosterone system, or the use of β-blockers can predispose to hyperkalemic states by interfering with the internal K^+ balance [3].

Renal Handling of Potassium

The ability of the kidneys to match the amount of K^+ excreted to the amount of K^+ ingested is essential for the homeostasis of the body. This external balance is mainly carried out by the kidneys since 90% of K^+ ingested is eliminated through the urine, while the remaining 10% is excreted in feces. For this reason, kidney failure is generally associated with hyperkalemia, due to the inability of the kidneys to adequately excrete potassium [2].

K^+ is freely filtered in the glomerulus and is reabsorbed almost entirely in the proximal tubule. The fine processes that regulate urinary K^+ excretion take place in the distal nephron, where complex mechanisms modulate the secretion and/or reabsorption of this ion (Fig. 3.1). Urine $[K^+]$ can exceed plasma $[K^+]$, due to the large K^+ secretory capacity of the distal nephron. Secretion is observed under conditions of normal or high K^+ intake. When K^+ content in the diet is very low the kidney is unable to fully suppress K^+ excretion, in contrast to what happens with Na^+. Therefore, in these conditions there may be a negative K^+ balance and hypokalemia develops [1].

As mentioned above, the proximal tubule is responsible for the reabsorption of most of the filtered K^+. This process occurs mainly via the paracellular route, either through passive diffusion and/or by solvent drag (Fig. 3.2a). Initially, the $[K^+]$ in the filtrate is equal to blood's $[K^+]$, but as water is reabsorbed in the proximal tubule the $[K^+]$ in the filtrate increases, establishing a chemical gradient that favors reabsorption of this ion through tight junctions of the proximal tubular cells. Furthermore, the transepithelial voltage becomes positive in the lumen of the later portions of the proximal tubule (segment S3). Thus, the electrical gradient also promotes K^+ reabsorption in this segment. Solvent drag, that is, the K^+ flow that accompanies the net movement of water through the paracellular pathway, also plays an important role in K^+ reabsorption [1].

Even though the proximal tubule does not transport K^+ via the transcellular route, this does not mean that it is not important in the cellular physiology of this segment. Like in most epithelia, proximal tubule cells have Na^+/K^+ ATPase in their basolateral membrane, whose activity establishes the concentration gradient necessary for the proper function of a wide variety of secondary active transporters, such as the Na^+/glucose or Na^+/amino acids cotransporters. The K^+ entering the cells through

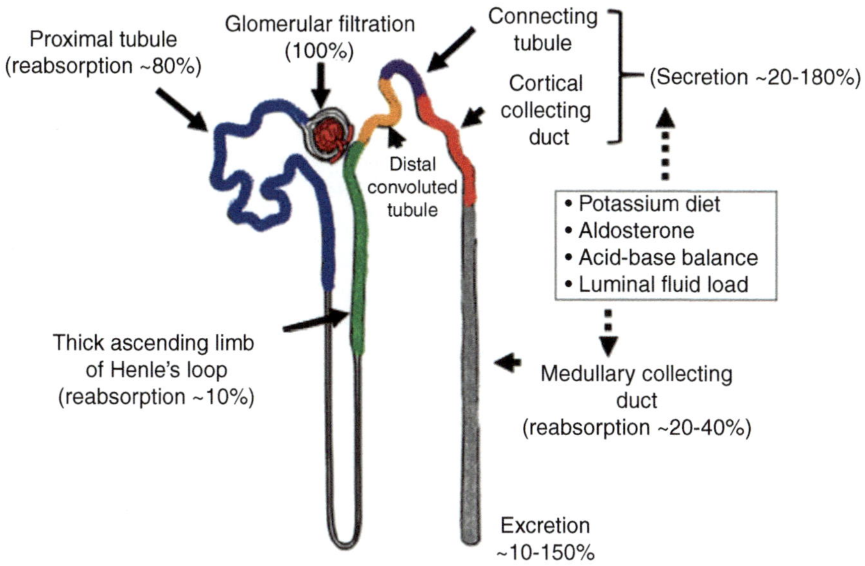

Fig. 3.1 K^+ renal handling. Various factors that modulate K^+ physiology in the distal nephron are indicated within the rectangle

the Na^+/K^+ ATPase is recycled to the interstitium through basolateral K^+ channels, as well as K^+/Cl^+ cotransporters (KCC) [4]. On the other hand, the apical permeability of K^+ in these cells is much lower than the basolateral permeability, perhaps due to the presence of K^+ ion channels that are closed under normal conditions and open only in response to changes in cell volume [5].

While K^+ reabsorption in the proximal tubule is paracellular and highly dependent on water transport, in the subsequent nephron segments K^+ transepithelial transport occurs mainly through the transcellular pathway and is carried out by a set of transporters, channels, and pumps that are regulated by diverse mechanisms.

K^+ transport in the thick ascending limb of Henle's loop occurs mainly through the furosemide-sensitive $Na^+/K^+/2Cl^-$ cotransporter (NKCC2) (Fig. 3.2b). Located in the apical membrane, this electroneutral cotransporter functions energized by the gradient established by the Na^+/K^+ ATPase. Na^+ and Cl^- ions transported by NKCC2 exit to the basolateral space through the Na^+/K^+ ATPase and Cl^- channels [6]. On the other hand, part of the K^+ introduced into the cell via NKCC2 is recycled into the tubular lumen by an inwardly rectifying ion channel, called ROMK. This K^+ recirculation is key to maintain NKCC2 function, since the $[K^+]$ in the lumen is relatively low, and this cotransporter requires all three ions to be present simultaneously to be translocated into the cell. The electrogenic output of K^+ through ROMK establishes a transepithelial, lumen-positive voltage that favors the paracellular reabsorption of cations in this segment of the nephron, such as Na^+, Ca^{2+}, and Mg^{2+}. Although K^+ could also be reabsorbed in this way, the renal medulla has a high interstitial $[K^+]$, which hinders this process [7, 8].

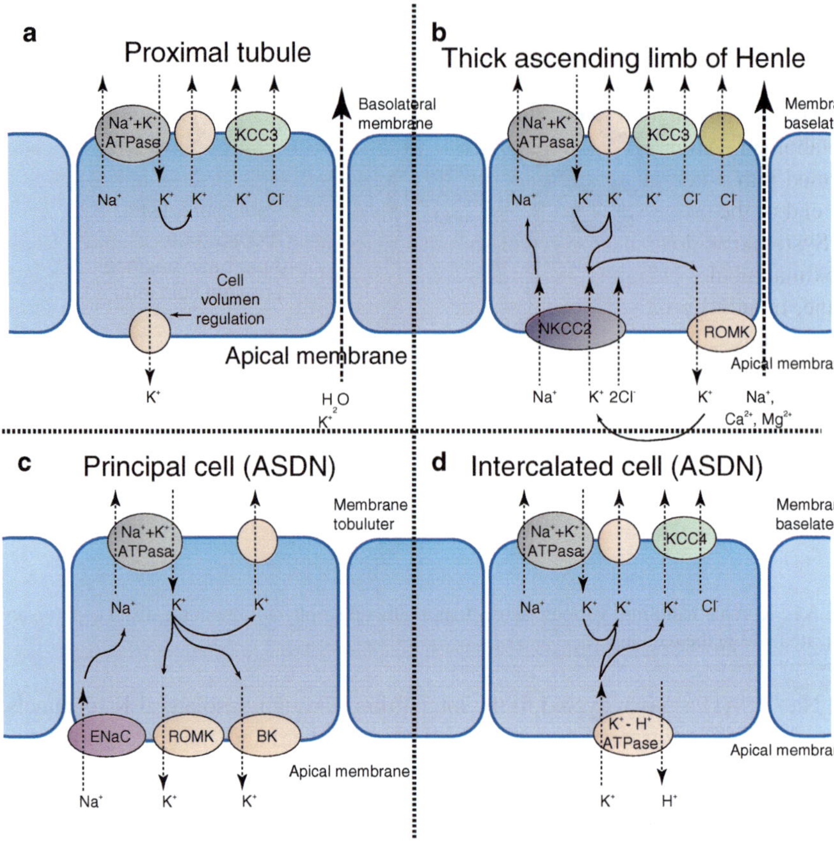

Fig. 3.2 K^+ transport mechanisms along the nephron, specifically in the proximal tubule (**a**), thick ascending limb of Henle's loop (**b**), principal cells of the aldosterone-sensitive nephron (ASDN) (**c**), and ASDN α-intercalated cells (**d**)

The basolateral membrane of the thick ascending limb of Henle's loop is also permeable to K^+ due to the presence of K^+ channels. Therefore, some of the K^+ that enters the cell via NKCC2 exits the cytoplasm to the basolateral fluid space through these K^+ channels. Through this mechanism, between 10 and 20% of the filtered K^+ is reabsorbed in this nephron segment. This amount varies according to physiological conditions. It has been reported that in some situations even K^+ secretion can occur [9]. Finally, the relationship between NKCC2 and renal K^+ handling is more complex, since cotransporter activity exerts an indirect effect on distal K^+ secretion, as will be explained later in this chapter.

The distal convoluted tubule does not play an important role in transepithelial K^+ transport [10]. Its main role is to carry out salt reabsorption through the thiazide-sensitive Na^+/Cl^- cotransporter (NCC). However, the activity of this cotransporter can indirectly modulate the distal mechanisms involved in K^+ secretion.

The connecting tubule (CNT) and the cortical collecting duct (CCT) constitute the aldosterone-sensitive distal nephron (ASDN). This segment contains a heterogeneous cell population, with 70% of principal cells responsible for K^+ secretion via the transcellular route. The remaining 30% are intercalated cells. Principal cells express the epithelial Na^+ channel (ENaC) in their apical membrane, as well as K^+ channels such as ROMK and BK that confer a high permeability to K^+. The entry of Na^+ through ENaC channels promotes the establishment of a lumen-positive transepithelial potential that favors apical K^+ extrusion through K^+ channels. Furthermore, Na^+ entry via ENaC is key to maintain basolateral Na^+/K^+ ATPase activity, thus allowing a constant entry of K^+ into the cell from the basolateral space fluid [1, 8]. The net result of this process is the electrogenic exchange of Na^+ for K^+ in the filtrate (Fig. 3.2c). On the other hand, α- and β-intercalated cells are responsible for reabsorbing K^+ through an H^+/K^+ ATPase expressed in their apical membrane (Fig. 3.2d). This mechanism operates mainly under K^+ deprivation conditions [11].

Finally, in the medullary collecting duct (MCD) K^+ reabsorption occurs through the H^+/K^+ ATPase, as well as through the paracellular route. Luminal $[K^+]$ in the MCD is high due to the active secretion of K^+ that takes place in previous segments. Also, water reabsorption occurs in this segment, particularly in the presence of antidiuretic hormone, and this further increases luminal $[K^+]$. Thus, the electrochemical gradient favors the passive diffusion of K^+ from the lumen to the interstitium [7, 8].

Factors that Regulate the Secretion of Potassium

The secretion of K^+ mediated by principal cells is modulated by a variety of factors. One of them is the amount of luminal flux that reaches this segment. With higher luminal flux, the luminal $[K^+]$ increases more slowly at a certain secretion rate [1, 8]. Additionally, BK apical channels are activated by high luminal flux, which increases the apical permeability to K^+ and, therefore, its secretion [12]. The effect of luminal flux on K^+ secretion may explain the well-known phenomenon that diuretics acting upstream of the connecting tubule (such as furosemide in the loop of Henle, or thiazides in the distal convoluted tubule) promote K^+ loss.

Likewise, genetic diseases such as Bartter's syndrome type I and Gitelman's syndrome, caused by loss-of-function mutations in the genes encoding NKCC2 and NCC, respectively, manifest with hypokalemia, in addition to other electrolyte abnormalities [6]. Interestingly, mutations in the gene encoding the ROMK channel are the cause of Bartter's syndrome type II, characterized by transient neonatal hyperkalemia, which disappears after one week of birth, probably due to compensation in the K^+ secretion process by BK channels. However, the absence of ROMK affects the NKCC2-mediated transport process in the loop of Henle, so hypokalemia may subsequently develop in these patients, in addition to hypotension, hypercalciuria, and nephrocalcinosis [7, 13].

On the other hand, familial hyperkalemic hypertension (also called Gordon's syndrome or pseudohypoaldosteronism type II), in which NCC activity is increased by mutations in genes involved in the regulation of this co-transporter, is characterized by a hyperkalemic state due to the inability of the connecting tubule to secrete potassium. In studies with murine models, it has been suggested that increased NCC activity promotes a remodeling effect of the nephron, specifically connecting tubule hypotrophy, which compromises K^+ secretion. This effect is reversible with the administration of hydrochlorothiazide for 3 days, indicating that NCC activity is an important modulator of the structure and physiology of ASDN [14].

Aldosterone is a steroid hormone produced in the *zona glomerulosa* of the adrenal gland. Its synthesis and release can be stimulated by angiotensin II in hypovolemic conditions or by increases in plasma $[K^+]$.

The mineralocorticoid receptor (MR) is a nuclear receptor and the target of aldosterone. However, it is also capable of binding cortisol, whose plasma concentration is much higher than that of aldosterone. Therefore, for a cell to respond to fluctuations in plasma aldosterone concentration, it must express an enzyme called 11-β-hydroxysteroid dehydrogenase type II (11-β-HSD2), which catalyzes the conversion of cortisol to cortisone that is unable to bind the MR. Principal cells in the ASDN express 11-β-HSD, and thus their MR is subject to modulation by aldosterone [1].

The occupation of MR by aldosterone allows its translocation to the nucleus, where it promotes the transcription of different genes, such as those that encode the Na^+/K^+ ATPase and, importantly, the kinase SGK1 [15]. The main function of this kinase is the phosphorylation and inactivation of the ubiquitin-ligase Nedd4-2, whose function is to promote the degradation of the ENaC channels. Therefore, SGK1 activity promotes an increase in the amount of ENaC and an increase in the electrogenic exchange of Na^+ by K^+, allowing the secretion of the latter [8].

The disruption of these mechanisms, by pharmacological inhibition or by genetic mutations, has an impact on K^+ secretion. Gain-of-function mutations in genes encoding the ENaC channel subunits prevent Nedd4-2 binding and, therefore, higher amounts of ENaC, promoting the hypokalemia observed in Liddle Syndrome [16]. In contrast, loss—of-function mutations in these same genes in pseudohypoaldosteronism type I (PHAI), or the pharmacological inhibition of ENaC by K^+-sparing diuretics (such as amiloride) are the cause of hyperkalemia. PHAI can also be caused by mutations in the MR gene or by its inhibition by antagonists such as spironolactone [17].

An interesting observation is that glycyrrhizinic acid, commonly found in licorice, has an inhibitory effect on 11-β-HSD2, allowing cortisol to bind to MR in the principal cells, thus causing hypokalemia. Likewise, loss-of-function mutations in the gene encoding this enzyme are the cause of apparent mineralocorticoid excess syndrome, characterized by a hypokalemic state and hypertension [18].

Although aldosterone plays an essential role in K^+ homeostasis, other mechanisms can regulate plasma K^+ levels to some extent. Different observations in diverse animal models with an absence of aldosterone [19], or with fixed levels of aldosterone, either by adrenalectomy or infusion [20], suggest that aldosterone-independent mechanisms participate in the regulation of K^+ secretion in response to changes in plasma [K^+]. One of these mechanisms is the modulation by plasma [K^+] of the NCC cotransporter in the distal convoluted tubule [21, 22]. In distal convoluted tubule cells, an increase in plasma [K^+] promotes membrane depolarization, which limits the efflux of Cl^- through the basolateral membrane [23]. The subsequent increase in intracellular [Cl^-] has an inhibitory effect on WNK4 kinase, which normally activates NCC through the SPAK/OSR1 kinases [24]. Furthermore, recent data suggest that a phosphatase may also respond to increased plasma [K^+] and promote NCC dephosphorylation and inactivation [25]. These processes increase the flow of Na^+ that reaches the ASDN and, therefore, the ability of principal cells to exchange Na^+ for K^+.

Finally, glucocorticoids play an indirect role in the response to K^+ loads, perhaps by regulating the glomerular filtration rate that affects the Na^+ flow reaching the ASDN. Supraphysiological concentrations of glucocorticoids can also increase K^+ secretion by directly binding to the MR, despite the presence of 11-β-HSD2 [1].

Relationship Between Renal Potassium Metabolism and Acid-Base Balance

Alterations of acid-base status affect body K^+ balance. In general, acidosis is associated with hyperkalemia, while alkalosis is associated with hypokalemia. This is because acid-base alterations affect intracellular storage of K^+, as well as renal excretion of K^+. Acidosis promotes the release of K^+ from the cells through different mechanisms: (1) Na^+/H^+ exchange and Na^+/HCO_3^- cotransport is inhibited; (2) this, in turn, results in a decrease in intracellular pH and a decrease in intracellular Na^+ concentration $[Na^+]_{IC}$; (3) intracellular acidosis decreases Na^+/K^+ ATPase activity and NKCC1 cotransporter activity; (4) furthermore, the decrease in $[Na^+]_{IC}$ also negatively affects the activity of Na^+/K^+ ATPase; (5) finally, the increase in $[H^+]_{IC}$ promotes displacement by H^+ ions of K^+ ions bound to non-diffusible intracellular anions (e.g., proteins), which promotes the exit of K^+ from the cells. All of this affects the intracellular storage of K^+. The opposite phenomena are observed during alkalosis and explain the hypokalemia associated with alkalosis [1, 26].

Regarding renal K^+ excretion, acute acidosis inhibits renal K^+ excretion through the following mechanisms. In principal cells of the nephron, the drop in basolateral fluid's pH leads to a decrease in intracellular pH, due to the inhibition of Na^+/H^+ exchange by the basolateral NHE1 exchanger. This, in turn, promotes the inhibition of various proteins involved in the K^+ secretory mechanism such as Na^+/K^+ ATPase, ENaC, ROMK, and BK channels. Furthermore, in α-intercalated cells the activity of H^+/K^+ ATPase is stimulated, thus, promoting the reabsorption of K^+ [26]. Alkalosis, in contrast, stimulates renal K^+ secretion, probably by affecting the same mechanisms in the opposite direction (Fig. 3.3a).

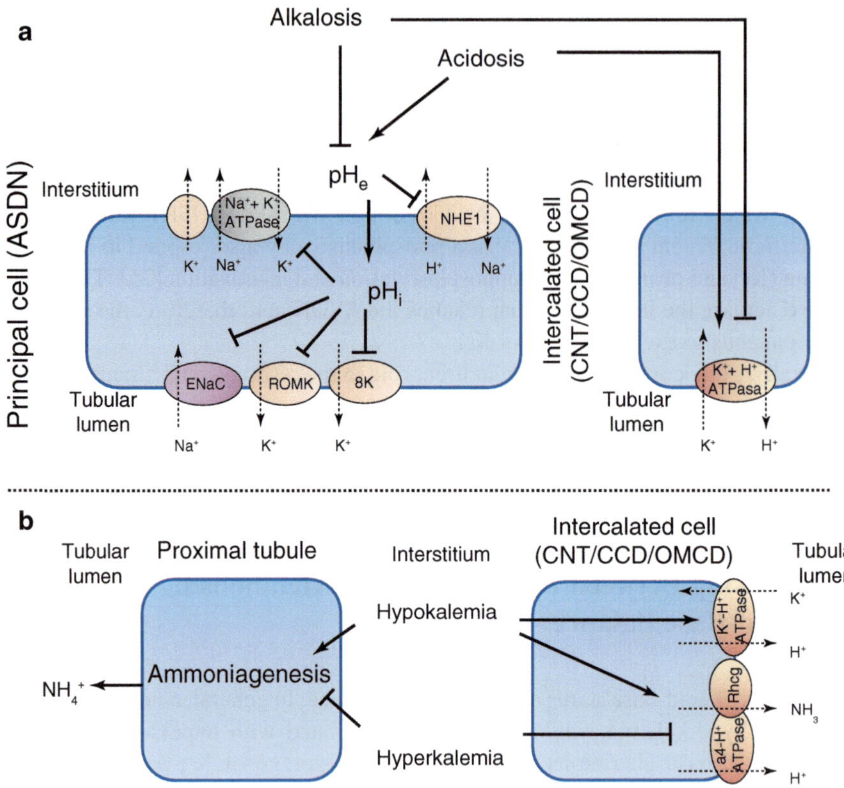

Fig. 3.3 Renal mechanisms are involved in the relationship between K^+ homeostasis and acid-base balance. Model of the effect of acid-base alterations on renal K^+ handling in the distal nephron (**a**). Model of the effect of plasma K^+ alterations on renal acid management by the proximal tubule and α-intercalated cells of the distal nephron (**b**)

In a chronic setting, however, acidosis promotes hypokalemia instead of hyperkalemia. For example, under conditions such as type 1 (distal) or type 2 (proximal) renal tubular acidosis, caused by defects in renal acid-base regulatory mechanisms, hypokalemia is usually observed. Changes in distal tubular flow produced in response to acid-base disturbances have been proposed to be responsible for this phenomenon. For example, metabolic acidosis inhibits proximal fluid reabsorption by inhibiting Na^+/K^+ ATPase activity in the cells of this segment, among other mechanisms. Consequently, the increase in distal tubular flow counteracts the negative effects of low pH on distal K^+ secretion mechanisms. In chronic conditions this mechanism predominates, producing hypokalemia. In chronic alkalosis, on the other hand, an increase in distal tubular flow is also observed that is caused by different mechanisms than those described for acidosis, and this enhances the loss of renal K^+ [26].

The opposite causal relationship also operates, that is, alterations in the K^+ balance affect the acid-base status of the organism. In general, hyperkalemia is associated with metabolic acidosis, while hypokalemia is associated with metabolic alkalosis. The exchange of K^+ for H^+, mainly in the skeletal muscle cells, due to the competition between K^+ and H^+ ions for binding sites in intracellular proteins is largely responsible for this phenomenon. For example, in the case of hypokalemia, the decrease in intracellular concentration of K^+ promotes the intracellular accumulation of H^+, thus promoting extracellular alkalinization.

In renal proximal tubular cells, intracellular acidification secondary to this phenomenon activates mechanisms involved in the excretion of H^+ and reabsorption of HCO_3^-, such as the apical Na^+/H^+ exchanger, as well as the basolateral co-transporter Na^+/HCO_3^- [26]. Furthermore, it increases the synthesis of NH_3 and excretion of NH_4^+, an important mechanism to increase the renal capacity to excrete H^+ ions. This latter effect is due to changes in the expression of proteins involved in ammonia synthesis, reversed when plasma [K^+] is normalized [27].

Finally, as mentioned above, during hypokalemia α-intercalated cells of the connecting tubule and collecting ducts promote the reabsorption of K^+ at the expense of secreting H^+ into the tubular lumen. Furthermore, hypokalemia also increases the membrane localization of the a4-H^+ATPase and the Rhcg protein, both responsible for the secretion of NH_4^+ in the intercalated cells of the collecting duct [27, 28]. These mechanisms also contribute to the development of hypokalemic alkalosis (Fig. 3.3b).

Again, the opposite mechanisms operate during hyperkalemia, explaining the association with metabolic acidosis. In fact, in the hyperkalemic subtypes of renal tubular acidosis, the primary alteration is normally a defect in renal K^+ secretion. As an example, in type 4 renal tubular acidosis, which is secondary to hypoaldosteronism, the decrease in aldosterone-stimulated K^+ secretion leads to hyperkalemia, which in turn causes acidosis. Likewise, in genetic diseases with alterations of distal K^+ secretion, as in type I and type II pseudo-hypoaldosteronisms, acidosis secondary to hyperkalemia is observed [26].

References

1. Boulpaep EL, Boron WF. Medical physiology. 3rd ed. Philadelphia: Elsevier; 2016.
2. Zacchia M, Abategiovanni ML, Stratigis S, Capasso G. Potassium: from physiology to clinical implications. Kidney Dis. 2016;2(2):72–9. https://doi.org/10.1159/000446268.
3. Palmer BF, Clegg DJ. Physiology and pathophysiology of potassium homeostasis. Adv Physiol Educ. 2016;40(4):480–90. https://doi.org/10.1152/advan.00121.2016.
4. Melo Z, Cruz-Rangel S, Bautista R, et al. Molecular evidence for a role for K+-Cl- cotransporters in the kidney. Am J Physiol Ren Physiol. 2013;305(10):1402–11. https://doi.org/10.1152/ajprenal.00390.2013.
5. Hebert SC, Desir G, Giebisch G, Wang W. Molecular diversity and regulation of renal potassium channels. Phisol Rev. 2005;3811:319–71. https://doi.org/10.1152/physrev.00051.2003.
6. Gamba G. Molecular physiology and pathophysiology of electroneutral cation-chloride cotransporters. Physiol Rev. 2005;85(2):423–93. https://doi.org/10.1152/physrev.00011.2004.

7. Welling PA, Ho K. A comprehensive guide to the ROMK potassium channel: form and function in health and disease. AJP Ren Physiol. 2009;297(4):F849–63. https://doi.org/10.1152/ajprenal.00181.2009.
8. Palmer LG, Schnermann J. Integrated control of na transport along the nephron. Clin J Am Soc Nephrol. 2015;10(4):676–87. https://doi.org/10.2215/CJN.12391213.
9. Wang B, Wen D, Li H, Wang-france J, Sansom SC. Net K+ secretion in the thick ascending limb of mice on a low-Na, high-K diet. Kidney Int. 2017;92(4):864–75. https://doi.org/10.1016/j.kint.2017.04.009.
10. Schnermann J, Steipe B, Briggs JP. In situ studies of distal convoluted tubule in rat. II. K secretion. Am J Physiol Physiol. 1987;252(6):F970–6. https://doi.org/10.1152/ajprenal.1987.252.6.F970.
11. Gumz ML, Lynch IJ, Greenlee MM, Cain BD, Wingo CS. The renal H+-K+-ATPases: physiology, regulation, and structure. Am J Physiol Ren Physiol. 2010;298(1):12–21. https://doi.org/10.1152/ajprenal.90723.2008.
12. Liu W, Xu S, Woda C, Kim P, Weinbaum S, Satlin LM. Effect of flow and stretch on the [Ca2+]i response of principal and intercalated cells in cortical collecting duct. Am J Physiol Ren Physiol. 2003;285(5 54-5):998–1012. https://doi.org/10.1152/ajprenal.00067.2003.
13. Finer G, Shalev H, Birk OS, et al. Transient neonatal hyperkalemia in the antenatal (ROMK defective) Bartter syndrome. J Pediatr. 2003;142(3):318–23. https://doi.org/10.1067/mpd.2003.100.
14. Grimm PR, Coleman R, Delpire E, Welling PA. Constitutively active SPAK causes hyperkalemia by activating NCC and remodeling distal tubules. J Am Soc Nephrol. 2017;28(9):2597–606. https://doi.org/10.1681/ASN.2016090948.
15. Valinsky WC, Touyz RM, Shrier A. Aldosterone, SGK1, and ion channels in the kidney. Clin Sci. 2018;132(2):173–83. https://doi.org/10.1042/CS20171525.
16. Palmer BF, Alpern RJ. Liddle's Syndrome. Am J Med. 1998;104(3):301–9. https://doi.org/10.1016/S0002-9343(98)00018-7.
17. Furgeson SB, Linas S. Mechanisms of type I and type II pseudohypoaldosteronism. J Am Soc Nephrol. 2010;21(11):1842–5. https://doi.org/10.1681/ASN.2010050457.
18. Ferrari P. The role of 11β-hydroxysteroid dehydrogenase type 2 in human hypertension. Biochim Biophys Acta Mol basis Dis. 2010;1802(12):1178–87. https://doi.org/10.1016/j.bbadis.2009.10.017.
19. Todkar A, Picard N, Loffing-Cueni D, et al. Mechanisms of renal control of potassium homeostasis in complete aldosterone deficiency. J Am Soc Nephrol. 2015;26(2):425–38. https://doi.org/10.1681/ASN.2013111156.
20. Young DB, Paulsen AW. Interrelated effects of aldosterone and plasma potassium on potassium excretion. Am J Physiol Ren Fluid Electrolyte Physiol. 1983;13(1) https://doi.org/10.1152/ajprenal.1983.244.1.f28.
21. Vallon V, Schroth J, Lang F, Kuhl D, Uchida S. Expression and phosphorylation of the Na+-Cl-cotransporter NCC in vivo is regulated by dietary salt, potassium, and SGK1. Am J Physiol Ren Physiol. 2009;297(3):F704–12. https://doi.org/10.1152/ajprenal.00030.2009.
22. Murillo-de-Ozores AR, Chávez-Canales M, de los Heros P, Gamba G, Castañeda-Bueno M. Physiological processes modulated by the chloride-sensitive WNK-SPAK/OSR1 kinase signaling pathway and the cation-coupled chloride cotransporters. Front Physiol. 2020;11(October):1–28. https://doi.org/10.3389/fphys.2020.585907.
23. Terker AS, Zhang C, McCormick JA, et al. Potassium modulates electrolyte balance and blood pressure through effects on distal cell voltage and chloride. Cell Metab. 2015;21(1):39–50. https://doi.org/10.1016/j.cmet.2014.12.006.
24. Bazua-Valenti S, Chavez-Canales M, Rojas-Vega L, et al. The effect of WNK4 on the Na+-Cl-cotransporter is modulated by intracellular chloride. J Am Soc Nephrol. 2015;26(8):1781–6. https://doi.org/10.1681/ASN.2014050470.

25. Penton D, Czogalla J, Wengi A, et al. Extracellular K + rapidly controls NaCl cotransporter phosphorylation in the native distal convoluted tubule by Cl − −dependent and independent mechanisms. J Physiol. 2016;594(21):6319–31. https://doi.org/10.1113/JP272504.
26. Aronson PS, Giebisch G. Effects of pH on potassium: new explanations for old observations. J Am Soc Nephrol. 2011;22(11):1981–9. https://doi.org/10.1681/ASN.2011040414.
27. Harris AN, Grimm PR, Lee H-W, et al. Mechanism of hyperkalemia-induced metabolic acidosis. J Am Soc Nephrol. 2018:ASN.2017111163. https://doi.org/10.1681/ASN.2017111163.
28. Han KH, Lee HW, Handlogten ME, et al. Effect of hypokalemia on renal expression of the ammonia transporter family members, Rh B glycoprotein and Rh C glycoprotein, in the rat kidney. Am J Physiol Ren Physiol. 2011;301(4):823–32. https://doi.org/10.1152/ajprenal.00266.2011.

Chapter 4
Genetic Origin of Renal Tubular Acidosis

Laura Escobar-Pérez and Rosa Vargas-Poussou

Introduction

Four types of renal tubular acidosis (RTA) have been described according to the chronological order in which the clinical cases were documented. Type I RTA corresponds to classic distal RTA or Albright's RTA described in the 1940s [1]. Type II RTA or proximal RTA was documented by Rodríguez-Soriano in the 1960s [2]. Type III RTA or mixed RTA was described in the 1970s [3]. Finally, Type IV RTA or hyperkalemic distal RTA was associated with hypo or pseudohypoaldosteronism [4].

In all types of RTA, hyperchloremic metabolic acidosis occurs with a normal blood anion gap (BAG), which is determined with the formula: $[Na^+] - ([Cl^-] + [HCO_3^-]) \leq 12$. When BAG is elevated, metabolic acidosis is normochloremic and may be secondary to an unmeasured endogenous anion (lactic acid, organic acids, ketone bodies, etc.), or the presence of an exogenous anion (acetylsalicylic acid, methanol or ethylene glycol poisonings). On the other hand, when BAG is normal, metabolic acidosis is secondary to the loss of bicarbonate, which can occur by intestinal losses (diarrhea, fistulas) or RTA: in proximal RTA bicarbonate is lost in the urine while in distal RTA bicarbonate is consumed in the

L. Escobar-Pérez (✉)
Department of Physiology, Faculty of Medicine, National Autonomous University of Mexico, Mexico City, Mexico

National Autonomous University of Mexico, Mexico City, Mexico

National System of Investigators, Mexico City, Mexico
e-mail: laurae@unam.mx

R. Vargas-Poussou
Département de Génetique, Hôpital Européen Georges Pompidou, Paris, France

R. Muñoz (ed.), *Renal Tubular Acidosis in Children*,
https://doi.org/10.1007/978-3-030-91940-5_4

plasma due to the inability to excrete hydrogen ions in the urine by the collecting ducts of the nephrons.

Hereditary kidney diseases show different frequencies, for example, polycystic kidney disease is the most common autosomal dominant alteration, and affects 1 in 1000 people. In contrast, the rest of the inherited kidney diseases occur infrecuently, which means that they impact less than 5 people per 10,000. In particular, RTA has a prevalence of approximately 1:100,000 in consanguineous marriages and less than 1:1 million in the rest of the population. Consequently, most physicians are unlikely to encounter a case of RTA during their medical practice.

RTA is a monogenic inherited disease. Gene mutations produce variable effects: premature stop codons, open reading frame shift, alternative RNA processing, or nucleotide point changes in codons, leading to changes in one or more amino acids, consequently, causing structural alterations in proteins, losing their function. Genes associated to RTA types in several populations are described below.

Autosomal Recessive Proximal RTA

This inherited form of RTA is due to mutations in SLC4A4 encoding the basolateral sodium/bicarbonate transporter (Na^+/HCO_3^-) NBCe1 of proximal tubular cells [5]. Alternative splicing of *SLC4A4* results in three isoforms, IA isoform (kNBCe1) is expressed in the proximal tubule, eye, and salivary glands. The other isoforms are expressed in pancreas, teeth, brain, and eye. In the eye, NBCe1 maintains corneal transparency, as well as ocular pressure. Consequently, mutations in *SLC4A4* explain its association with ocular manifestations such as band keratopathy, cataracts, and glaucoma (Table 4.1). Other extra-renal manifestations are dental enamel defects, mental retardation, basal ganglia calcification, migraine, hyperthyroidism, and increased amylase without pancreatitis [6].

Autosomal Dominant Proximal RTA

In 1977, Luis Brenes documented the case of a family in which nine members presented proximal RTA in a "pure" form better known as isolated proximal RTA without ocular involvement. They had hyperchloremic metabolic acidosis with normal plasma creatinine values and the ability to acidify urine, and were asymptomatic. The only feature was short stature [7] despite lack of hypercalciuria. To date, only two families with isolated proximal RTA have been described [8]. Several candidate genes have been analyzed, but the associated gene has not yet been identified (Table 4.2).

Table 4.1 Type of RTA, transmission, age of presentation, clinical and biology, protein involved, Gen/locus/OMIM

Proximal, recessive, first months, growth delay
Eye abnormalities (banded keratopathy, cataracts, and glaucoma)
Mental retardation, brain calcifications
Defects in tooth enamel
Increased serum amylases
Severe metabolic acidosis
Hypokalemia, Na^+/HCO_3^- or NBCe1 exchanger; SLC4A4/4q21 /604278
Dominant protein? Gen/locus/OMIM ? /? / 179830
Distal Dominant
(complete or incomplete)
Adult/adolescence
Lithiasis and/or nephrocalcinosis
Muscular weakness
Osteomalacia/osteoporosis
Moderate metabolic acidosis
Hypokalemia, hypocitraturia, hypercalciuria
Exchanger
Cl^-/HCO_3^- or AE1. Gen/locus/OMIM: SLC4A1/17q21-22/179800
Recessive *,
Childhood. Hemolytic anemia. Metabolic acidosis. Growth-retarded.
Exchanger: Cl−/HCO3− or AE1. Gen/locus/OMIM: SLC4A1 / 17q21-22 / 611590
Recessive
First months. Growth delay.
Vomiting, dehydration
Early nephrocalcinosis
Sensorineural deafness
Rickets
Severe metabolic acidosis
Hypokalemia, hypocitraturia, hypercalciuria.
Genes/locus/OMIM: V-ATPase subunit B1, ATP6V1B1/ 2p13/267300; V-ATPase a4 subunit, ATP6V0A4 / 7q33-34 / 602722
Mixed, proximal and distal. Recessive. First months /childhood. Carbonic anhydrase II or AC II. Gene/locus/OMIM: CA2 / 8q22 / 259730

*Described only in Southwest Asia. The numbers in the circles correspond to the location of the proteins involved in Fig. 4.1.

Fanconi Syndrome with Proximal RTA

In proximal RTA associated with Fanconi syndrome, in addition to hypokalemia and hyperchloremic acidosis, patients have generalized proximal tubular defects; they lose sodium, phosphate, glucose, low molecular weight proteins, amino acids, etc.

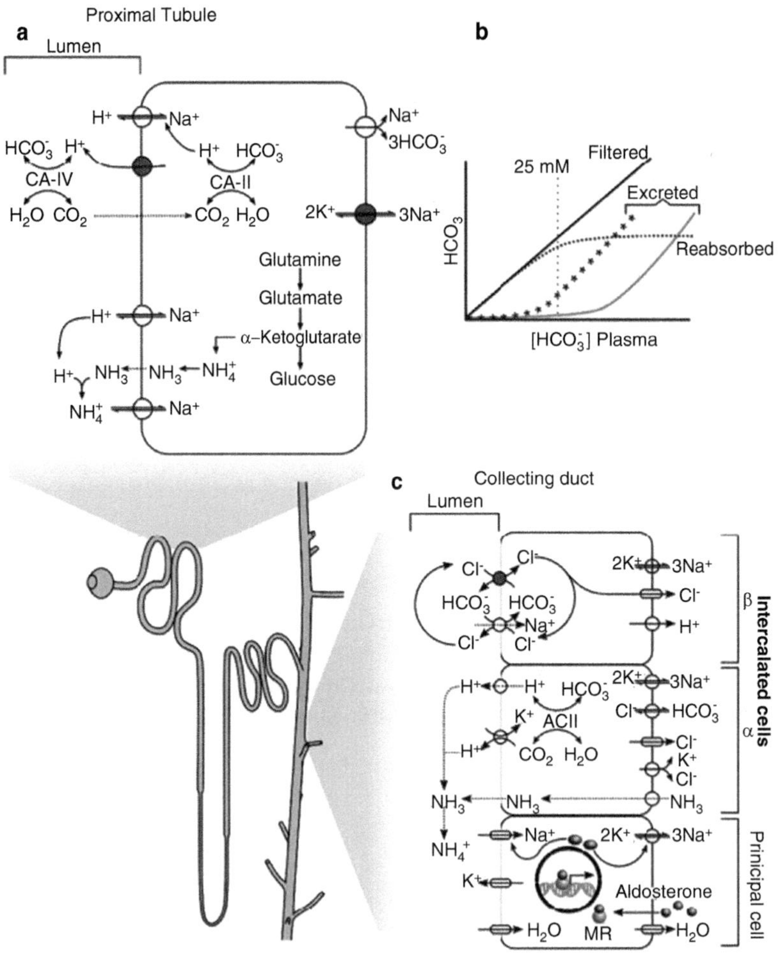

Fig. 4.1 Mechanisms of urinary acidification. (**a**) Schematic representation of a proximal tubular cell; filtered bicarbonate is recovered in this segment; glutamine degradation, ammonium, and bicarbonate synthesis are performed. The transport systems involved in proximal bicarbonate reabsorption include Na^+/H^+ exchanger (NHE3) and H^+-ATPase (V-ATPase), which secrete hydrogen ion (H^+) into the urine; carbonic anhydrase IV (AC-IV) accelerates the dehydration of carbonic acid (H_2CO_3); carbonic anhydrase II (AC-II) is cytosolic and catalyzes the hydration of CO_2; finally, the sodium bicarbonate transporter ($NaHCO_3$, NBCe1), guarantees the reabsorption of bicarbonate due to its location in the basolateral membrane. (**b**) Representation of filtered (black), excreted (gray), and reabsorbed (dots) bicarbonate. When plasma bicarbonate increases (metabolic alkalosis), its excretion in the urine is observed (gray line). The curve with asterisks corresponds to the bicarbonate load excreted in a patient with proximal RTA; a decreased threshold of plasma bicarbonate concentration is observed. (**c**) Representation of α/β intercalated cells and principal cells of the collecting duct. Intercalated H^+ secreting cells are type α. Hydrogen ion secretion is carried out by H^+-ATPase (V-ATPase) and ATPase K^+-H^+ pumps on the apical membrane. Reabsorption of sodium (Na^+) by principal cells generates a negative transepithelial gradient in the lumen that favors H^+ secretion. In the cytosol, carbonic anhydrase AC II catalyzes the hydration of CO_2; the bicarbonate generated is reabsorbed through the basolateral exchanger AE1. NH3 transport by RhBG and RhCG channels is depicted

Table 4.2 Hyperkalemic Type IV renal tubular acidosis

Primary congenital hypoaldosteronism. Suprarenal hyperplasia (21-hydroxylase, 3-β-OH dehydrogenase, or desmolase deficiency)
Acquired Addison's disease
Isolated mineralocorticoid deficiency
Acquired Hyporeninemic hypoaldosteronism: Diabetic nephropathy, interstitial Nephritis, prostaglandin inhibitors
Pseudo-hypoaldosteronism (mineralocorticoid resistance). Congenital. Type I (with salt loss and hypotension)
Autosomal dominant or renal form: mutations in the mineralocorticoid receptor gene (MLR or NR3C2)
Autosomal recessive or generalized form: mutations in three genes of ENaC sodium channel subunits (SCNN1A, SCNN1B, and SCNN1G)
Pseudo-hypoaldosteronism Congenital Type II (with sodium retention and hypertension): Gordon syndrome
Pseudo-hypoaldosteronism Autosomal dominant: mutations in the genes of two kinases (WNK1 and WNK4) or the ubiquitin ligase complexes KLHL3 - cullin 3 (KLHL3 and CUL3)
Pseudo-hypoaldosteronism Autosomal recessive: mutations in the KLHL3 gene
Pseudo-hypoaldosteronism Acquired.: Tubulointerstitial nephritis and obstructive uropathy

The exome (genome formed by exons) of a Mexican adolescent with Fanconi syndrome and isolated proximal RTA was recently analyzed. Until now, it is the only case reported in the literature [9]. Two heterozygous variants were identified in the SLC26A1 sulfate/oxalate exchanger. The glomerulus filters sulfates and oxalates freely; sulfates are reabsorbed in the proximal tubule, in contrast, oxalates are excreted by the luminal membranes of this segment. The SLC26A1 exchanger is located in the basolateral membrane of the proximal tubule and participates in the efflux of sulfate toward the interstitium by exchange with oxalate, which is excreted in the apical membrane by the SLC26A6 transporter [10]. Mice in which SLC26A1 expression is suppressed develop urolithiasis, hyperoxaluria, increased blood oxalates, decreased blood sulfates, and increased urine excretion of sulfates, as well as hepatotoxicity [11]. However, mutations in the SLC26A1 exchanger in humans and their consequences are not known.

In collaboration with the Seth Alper group, heterozygous variants in the SLC26A1 gene (C41W and A56T) were identified in the Mexican patient. However, these variants did not lose their function in *Xenopus* frog oocytes [9]. No mutations were found in other transporters involved in Fanconi syndrome such as the phosphate transporter NaPiIIa/SLC34A1 [12] or the glucose transporter GLUT2/SLC5A2 of Fanconi-Bickel syndrome [13]. Therefore, the molecular origin of Fanconi syndrome accompanied by isolated proximal RTA is unknown, except that it is autosomal recessive.

Distal RTA

Determination of urinary anion gap (UAG) is used to differentiate distal RTA from metabolic acidosis of any other etiology. In this case, the undetermined cation is ammonium (NH_4^+). Ammonium excretion is decreased when the result is positive, thus ruling out other possibilities of metabolic acidosis with a different etiology. In distal RTA, acid-secreting intercalated cells do not eliminate the acid load (ammonium and phosphate diacid) in the urine. Most of the patients studied have mutations in three proteins present in these cells: the chloride/bicarbonate exchanger AE1 (*SCL4A1*) and two subunits of the V-ATPase (V-H^+ATPase): a4 (*ATP6V0A4*) and B1 (*ATP6V1B1*). However, autosomal dominant distal RTA is due to mutations only in AE1, whereas autosomal recessive distal RTA is explained by mutations in AE1 or the a4 and B1 subunits of V-ATPase.

Distal RTA comprises 80% of the genetic forms. Still, its prevalence is low, approximately 1:1 million, and in consanguineous marriages approximately 1:100,000 [14]. Knowledge of the genetic bases of this entity has greatly contributed to the understanding of the molecular mechanisms involved in the acid-base balance regulated by the kidney.

In conclusion, the autosomal recessive distal RTA comprises a heterogeneous group of genes (five) and only one *(SLC4A1),* in the autosomal dominant RTA.

Autosomal Dominant Distal RTA

In the autosomal dominant distal RTA, one of the parents suffers the disease; it appears in late childhood or adulthood and is due to mutations in the *SLC4A1* gene,: the anion exchanger 1 (AE1).

Michael Tanner [15] from the University of Bristol and Fiona Karet [16] from the Cambridge Institute of Medical Research were the first to identify families with mutations in the *SLC4A1* gene. Mutations in AE1 are always heterozygous. AE1 is also expressed in erythrocytes, so the loss of its function produces hereditary spherocytosis and ovalocytosis in addition to distal RTA. It is noteworthy that the kidney-specific AE1 isoform is shorter: it does not have the first 65 amino acids of the amino-terminal AE1 of the erythrocyte. Consequently, in the autosomal dominant distal RTA, renal function is only affected when mutations in AE1 are located in the transmembrane domain or the carboxyl-terminal [17].

Autosomal Recessive Distal RTA Is Heterogeneous

In autosomal recessive distal RTA, parents do not have the disease, they are only carriers. In this case, the signs appear during pregnancy (polyhydramnios). In the infant, the clinical manifestations appear in the first months of life.

Early genetic studies of autosomal recessive distal RTA revealed mutations in the following genes: *SLC4A1* [18] and *ATP6V0A4, ATP6V1B1* [19–23]. Fiona Karet's group pioneered lineage studies in families with autosomal recessive distal RTA [21]. The majority of the families that were analyzed were from Turkey and Arabia, among consanguineous marriages. The age of children with autosomal recessive distal RTA who participated in the study ranged from 1 month to 3 years; all presented nephrocalcinosis and hypercalciuria and more than 50% sensorineural deafness, because V-ATPase is also expressed in the ciliated cells of the inner ear. These findings further confirmed that the enzyme H-K-ATPase, present in the α-intercalated cells, cannot compensate for the lack of functionality of the V-ATPase.

a4 and B1 subunits of V-ATPase are located in the kidney and inner ear; a4 subunit is present in the Vo domain and B1 subunit of V1 domain and, the genes are *ATP6V0A4* and *ATP6B1V1*, respectively [22]. Mutations in any of these genes are responsible for the decrease or loss of V-ATPase of the inner ear, which participates in the homeostasis of the endolymph pH, essential for normal hearing. In addition to nervous deafness, an expansion of the vestibular aqueduct frequently occurs [24].

In general, mutations of the B1 subunit are associated with hearing loss in childhood; patients with mutations in a4 subunit have moderate and late deafness in adolescence. However, some studies have concluded that the age of onset and the severity of the hearing loss are independent of the V-ATPase gene [23].

In dizygotic twins of different sex with autosomal recessive distal RTA and the same mutation in intron 6:, only one developed deafness; the cause of this is not known [25].

Autosomal Recessive Distal RTA Has Been Documented in Several Racial Groups

Mutations in the *ATP6V1B1* and *ATP6V0A4* genes have been described in families of diverse origin, such as Arabic, Turkish, Spanish [22]; African [23], Greek [26], Albanian and Italian [27], Tunisian [28], Japanese [29], Chinese [30–33], Brazilian [34], Mexican [35], and Korean [36]; and only mutations in *ATP6V1B1* in families of Spanish origin [25], Iranian [37], Kosovar [38], and Hindu [39]. The number of patients analyzed is variable due to the difficulty of finding them.

Unfortunately, in Mexico, several pediatricians associate failure to thrive to RTA [40], and diagnosis is made without any of the parameters established for this syndrome.

We performed the genetic analysis of nine Mexican patients [35]. Mutations were identified in the *ATP6V1B1* and *ATP6V0A4* genes; three cases were homozygous variants in *ATP6V1B1*, a change in the reading frame, a point mutation in exon 10 (p.Pro346Arg), and an unreported mutation in intron 5. Three patients were homozygous for an unreported point mutation (p.Arg743Trp) and a known one (p.Asp411Tyr) in the *ATP6V0A4* gene. Three cases were compound heterozygotes:

one case had two new mutations (p.Val52Metfs * 25) and a deletion of exons 18-21; two patients showed the point mutation p.Asp411Tyr and a second mutation, p.Arg184X and c.1691 + 2dup, respectively.

FOXI1 Transcription Factor

A recent study with three patients from two unrelated inbred families identified homozygous point mutations (p.L146F and p.R213P) in the transcription factor FOXI1, which regulates the expression of transporters AE1, AE4 [41] and subunits of V-ATPase B1, a4, A, and E2 [42]. Clinical features were early deafness and distal RTA. Mutations in the transcription factor FOXI1 inhibit their binding to the DNA of these genes, therefore, they are not expressed.

Autosomal Dominant Distal RTA

Autosomal dominant distal RTA is diagnosed in the majority of cases between adolescence and adulthood, followed by nephritic colic or the presence of nephrocalcinosis and osteoporosis, or is manifested by symptomatic hypokalemia (muscle weakness). Hypokalemia and hyperchloremic acidosis are less severe than those manifested in the recessive forms of distal RTA. In some patients, metabolic acidosis is not present, but the defect in the secretion of hydrogen ions is detected with a urinary acidification test; this form of RTA is called "incomplete distal RTA".

This dominant form of transmission is due to mutations in the heterozygous state of the *SLC4A1* gene. There are two AE1 isoforms: one isoform is expressed only in erythrocytes (also known as band 3), and the renal isoform is shorter (it does not have the first 65 amino acids of the amino acid terminal). Mutations of this gene are also associated with spherocytosis and ovalocytosis in Southeast Asia (OSA) (SEA). In OSA, erythrocytes are oval and most patients are asymptomatic; occasionally, they have mild symptoms such as paleness, jaundice, anemia, and gallstones.

Ovalocytosis is a red cell morphological abnormality caused by the 27 base pair deletion at codons 400 to 408 of the gene. The most frequent mutations found in unrelated families are G701D, A858D, and ΔV850, while other mutations have been described in some families [18, 43, 44]. In Thailand, mutations in the SLC4A1 gene explain 50% of distal RTA [44], and no mutations in the *ATP6V1B1* and *ATP6V0A4* have been found.

Curiously, mutations responsible for hematological changes are different from those involved in distal RTA. AE1 mutations in distal RTA lead to retention of the protein in the endoplasmic reticulum or abnormal targeting of the protein to the apical membrane of the α-intercalated acid-secreting cells. The homozygous Δ400-408 deletion and heterozygotes composed of four mutations (R602H, G701D, ΔV850, and A858D) develop ovalocytosis and distal RTA [45].

Dominant distal RTA develops in adulthood and its diagnosis and treatment are commonly delayed, as is the case of a male with a history of paralysis, moderate hypokalemia, and normal blood pH with hypercalciuria. The father presented the same clinical picture. Both were identified as having a heterozygous mutation (c.1162C > T, p.Arg388Cys) in exon 11 of SLC4A1 [46].

Recently, we performed the genetic analysis of a Mexican family with autosomal dominant distal RTA. It was a heterozygous variation (deletion in exon 20 of *SLC4A1*; https://doi.org/10.1016/j.nefro.2021.09.014) in two brothers (girl and boy) and their mother; the father did not have the mutation. This finding is of interest because it demonstrates the first case of autosomal dominant distal RTA in Latin America.

Autosomal Recessive Distal RTA Due to *SLC4A1*

Mutations in the *SLC4A1* gene encoding the chloride/bicarbonate anion exchanger AE1 (Cl^-/HCO_3^-) also produce autosomal recessive distal RTA. So far, more than 10 mutations of the *SLC4A1* gene produce RTA, in addition to ovalocytosis or spherocytosis [45]. Mutations in AE1 have been found mostly in the Asian tropical population of Thailand, Malaysia, the Philippines, and New Guinea [44]. Distal RTA cases in Asia are an example of natural selection because they are resistant to malaria.

Families with autosomal dominant and recessive distal RTA in the *SLC4A1* gene have been reported in China. In a family with distal RTA of autosomal recessive origin, both parents were carriers of the mutations: G494S and G701D [36, 46–48].

To date, more than 30 mutations in *SLC4A1* and *ATP6V1B1* and 50 mutations in *ATP6V0A4* have been published and all affect the traffic of the AE1 exchanger to the basolateral membrane of the α-intercalated cells and the synthesis or activity of V-ATPase (https://www.HGMD.CF.AC.UK/, www.ensembl.org and www.hgmd.org; [49]). Most of the mutations are homozygous and exceptionally heterozygous compounds.

WDR72

Three children with distal RTA of unknown origin were recently reported in a Thai family. Two pathogenic variations were found: ([p.R593G *] and [p.L841Q] in the protein called "72 tryptophan-aspartate repeat domain" (WDR72) [50]. WDR72 is an intracellular protein with two beta-sheets and one alpha-solenoid at its C-terminus.

WDR72 is a domain of vesicle proteins involved in the deformation mediating complexes of membranes that regulate intracellular trafficking [51]. However, the function of WDR72 is not yet known.

Mixed Renal Tubular Acidosis (Type III)

This form of RTA was discovered in 1972 by William Sly's group in the United States. Mixed RTA combines proximal bicarbonate reabsorption and distal hydrogen secretion defects. Autosomal recessive transmission mixed RTA occurs with osteopetrosis and calcifications in the brain and is associated with mutations in the carbonic anhydrase AC II gene. This enzyme participates in the proximal and α-intercalated cells in the reabsorption of bicarbonate and secretion of hydrogen ions, respectively, which explain the mixed nature of this RTA. AC II is also expressed in osteoclasts, where it plays an important role in acid secretion and bone resorption; its absence is responsible for the increase in bone density and fragility of osteopetrosis and is associated with calcifications in the brain and mental retardation. Conductive deafness and blindness may be present as side effects of bone compression [52]. Genetic analysis was performed for the first time with 12 unrelated families from: United States, Saudi Arabia, France, Belgium, and Kuwait [53]. AC II deficiency is most common in the Middle East of the Arabian peninsula having the junctional mutation of exon 2-intron 2 of the AC II gene [54].

Association between primary pulmonary hypertension and AC II deficiency has also been suggested [55].

Hyperkalemic RTA (Type IV)

The coexistence of hyperchloremic metabolic acidosis and hyperkalemia indicates a generalized collecting duct dysfunction. The main causes are summarized in Table 4.3, corresponding to the abnormalities associated with hypo or pseudo-hypoaldosteronism. Under these conditions, lack of aldosterone or resistance to its action is responsible for a defect in distal sodium reabsorption, which prevents the generation of the transepithelial gradient necessary for potassium and hydrogen ion secretion.

In conclusion, genetic studies have made an extraordinary contribution to the understanding of the complexity of the mechanisms underlying the renal acid-base balance. Cases of hereditary RTA that have not been explained with the genes known up to now, constitute a challenge in the identification of new molecular players involved in acid-base homeostasis in the kidney.

Table 4.3 Hyperkalemic Type IV renal tubular acidosis

Primary congenital hypoaldosteronism, suprarenal hyperplasia (21-hydroxylase, 3-β-OH dehydrogenase or desmolase deficiency)
Acquired Addison's disease
Isolated mineralocorticoid deficiency
Acquired Hyporeninemic Hypoaldosteronism: Diabetic Nephropathy, Interstitial Nephritis, Prostaglandin Inhibitors
Pseudo-hypoaldosteronism (mineralocorticoid resistance) Congenital Type I (with salt loss and hypotension)
Autosomal dominant or renal form: mutations in the mineralocorticoid receptor gene (MLR or NR3C2)
Autosomal recessive or generalized form: mutations in the genes of one of the three ENaC sodium channel subunits (SCNN1A, SCNN1B, and SCNN1G)
Pseudohypoaldosteronism Type II (with sodium retention and hypertension). Gordon syndrome
Autosomal dominant: mutations in the genes of two kinases (WNK1 and WNK4) or of the ubiquitin ligase complexes KLHL3 - cullin 3 (KLHL3 and CUL3)
Autosomal recessive: mutations in the KLHL3 gene
Acquired tubulointerstitial nephritis and obstructive uropathy

References

1. Albright F, Burnett CH, Parsons W, Reifenstein EC, Roos A. Osteomalacia and late rickets: various etiologies met in the United States with emphasis on that resulting from a specific form of renal acidosis, the therapeutic indications for each etiological sub-group, and the relationship between osteomalacia and Milkman's syndrome. Medicine. 1946;25:399–479.
2. Rodriguez Soriano J, Boichis H, Stark H, Edelmann CM Jr. Proximal renal tubular acidosis. A defect in bicarbonate reabsorption with normal urinary acidification. Pediatr Res. 1967;1:81–98.
3. Guibaud P, Larbre F, Freycon MT, Genoud J. Osteopetrosis and renal tubular acidosis. 2 cases of this association in a sibship. Arch Fr Pediatr. 1972;29:269–86.
4. Karet FE. Inherited distal renal tubular acidosis. J Am Soc Nephrol. 2002;13:2178–84.
5. Kurtz I, Zhu Q. Proximal renal tubular acidosis mediated by mutations in NBCe1-A: unraveling the transporter's structure-functional properties. Front Physiol. 2013;4:350 (1-11).
6. Igarashi T, Sekine T, Inatomi J, Seki G. Unraveling the molecular pathogenesis of isolated proximal renal tubular acidosis. J Am Soc Nephrol. 2002;13:2171–7.
7. Brenes LG, Brenes JN, Hernandez MM. Familial proximal renal tubular acidosis. A distinct clinical entity. Am J Med. 1977;63:244–52.
8. Lemann J Jr, Adams ND, Wilz DR, Brenes LG. Acid and mineral balances and bone in familial proximal renal tubular acidosis. Kidney Int. 2000;58:1267–77.
9. Wu M, Heneghan JF, Vandorpe DH, Escobar LI, Wu BL, Alper SL. Extracellular Cl- regulates human SO42−/anion exchanger SLC26A1 by altering pH sensitivity of anion transport. Pflügers Arch-Eur J Physiol. 2016;468:1311–32.
10. Markovich D. Physiological roles of renal anion transporters NaS1 and Sat1. Am J Physiol Renal Physiol. 2011;300:F1267–70.
11. Dawson PA, Russell CS, Lee S, McLeay SC, van Dongen JM, Cowley DM, Clarke LA, Markovich D. Urolithiasis and hepatotoxicity are linked to the anion transporter Sat1 in mice. J Clin Invest. 2010;120:706–12.

12. Magen D, Berger L, Coady MJ, Ilivitzki A, Militianu D, Tieder M, Selig S, Lapointe JY, Zelikovic I, SkoreckiK. A loss-of-function mutation in NaPi-IIa and renal Fanconi's syndrome. N Engl J Med. 2010;362:1102–9.
13. Santer R, Calado J. Familial renal glucosuria and SGLT2: from a mendelian trait to a therapeutic target. Clin J Am Soc Nephrol. 2010;5:133–41.
14. Escobar Pérez LI, Mejía N, Gil H, y Santos F. La acidosis tubular renal distal (ATRD): una enfermedad hereditaria rara en la que no se puede eliminar la carga ácida. Nefrologia. 2013;33:289–96.
15. Bruce LJ, Cope DL, Jones GK, Schofield AE, Burley M, Povey S, Unwin RJ, Wrong O, Tanner MJ. Familial distal renal tubular acidosis is associated with mutations in the red cell anion exchanger (Band 3, AE1) gene. J Clin Invest. 1997;100:1693–707.
16. Karet FE, Gainza FJ, Gÿory AZ, Unwin RJ, Wrong O, Tanner MJ, Nayir A, Alpay H, Santos F, Hulton SA, Bakkaloglu A, Ozen S, Cunningham MJ, di Pietro A, Walker WG, Lifton RP. Mutations in the chloride-bicarbonate exchanger gene AE1 cause autosomal dominant but not autosomal recessive distal renal tubular acidosis. Proc Natl Acad Sci U S A. 1998;95:6337–42.
17. Alper SL. Molecular physiology and genetics of Na-independent SLC4 anion exchangers. J Exp Biol. 2009;212:1672–83.
18. Tanphaichitr VS, Sumboonnanonda A, Ideguchi H, Shayakul C, Brugnara C, Takao M, et al. Novel AE1 mutations in recessive distal renal tubular acidosis. Loss-of-function is rescued by glycophorin A. J Clin Invest. 1998;102:2173–9.
19. Smith AN, Skaug J, Choate KA, Nayir A, Bakkaloglu A, Ozen S, et al. Mutations in ATP6N1B, encoding a new kidney vacuolar proton pump 116-kD subunit, cause recessive distal renal tubular acidosis with preserved hearing. Nat Genet. 2000;26:71–5.
20. Karet FE, Finberg KE, Nelson RD, Nayir A, Mocan H, Sanjad SA, et al. Mutations in the gene encoding B1 subunit of H+-ATPase cause renal tubular acidosis with sensorineural deafness. Nat Genet. 1999a;21:84–90.
21. Karet FE, Finberg KE, Nayir A, Bakkaloglu A, Ozen S, Hulton SA, et al. Localization of a gene for autosomal recessive distal renal tubular acidosis with normal hearing (rdRTA2) to 7q33-34. Am J Hum Genet. 1999b;65:1656–65.
22. Karet FE. Mechanisms in hyperkalemic renal tubular acidosis. J Am Soc Nephrol. 2009;20:251–4.
23. Vargas-Poussou R, Houillier P, Le Pottier N, Strompf L, Loirat C, Baudouin V, et al. Genetic investigation of autosomal recessive distal renal tubular acidosis: evidence for early sensorineural hearing loss associated with mutations in the ATP6V0A4 gene. J Am Soc Nephrol. 2006;17:1437–43.
24. Yashima T, Noguchi Y, Kawashima Y, Rai T, Ito T, Kitamura K. Novel atp6v1b1 mutations in distal renal tubular acidosis and hearing loss. Acta Otolaryngol. 2010;130:1002–8.
25. Gil H, Santos F, García E, Alvarez MV, Ordóñez FA, Málaga S, Coto E. Distal RTA with nerve deafness: clinical spectrum and mutational analysis in five children. Pediatr Nephrol. 2007;22:825–8.
26. Feldman M, Prikis M, Athanasiou Y, Elia A, Pierides A, Deltas DD. Molecular investigation and long-term clinical progress in Greek Cypriot families with recessive distal renal tubular acidosis and sensorineural deafness. Clin Genet. 2006;69(2):135–44.
27. Andreucci E, Bianchi B, Carboni I, Lavoratti G, Mortilla M, Fonda C, Bigozzi M, Genuardi M, Giglio S, Pela I. Inner ear abnormalities in four patients with dRTA and SNHL: clinical and genetic heterogeneity. Pediatr Nephrol. 2009;24:2147–53.
28. Elhayek D, Perez de Nanclares G, Chouchane S, Hamami S, Mlika A, Troudi M, Leban N, Ben Romdane W, Gueddiche MN, El Amri F, Mrabet S, Ben Chibani J, Castaño L, Haj Khelil A, Ariceta G. Molecular diagnosis of distal renal tubular acidosis in Tunisian patients: proposed algorithm for Northern Africa populations for the ATP6V1B1, ATP6V0A4 and SCL4A1 genes. BMC Med Genet. 2013;14:119 (1-10).

29. Miura K, Sekine T, Takahashi K, Takita J, Harita Y, Ohki K, Park MJ, Hayashi Y, Tajima A, Ishihara M, Hisano M, Murai M, Igarashi T. Mutational analyses of the ATP6V1B1 and ATP6V0A4 genes in patients with primary distal renal tubular acidosis. Nephrol Dial Transplant. 2013;28:2123–30.
30. Gao Y, Xu Y, Li Q, Lang Y, Dong Q, Shao L. Mutation analysis and audiological assessment in six Chinese children with primary distal renal tubular acidosis. Ren Fail. 2014;36:1226–32.
31. Zhang C, Ren H, Shen P, Xu Y, Zhang W, Wang W, Li X, Ma Y, Chen N. Clinical evaluation of Chinese patients with primary distal renal tubular acidosis. Intern Med. 2015;54:725–30.
32. Zhao X, Lu J, Gao Y, Wang X, Lang Y, Shao L. Novel compound heterozygous ATP6V1B1 mutations in a Chinese child patient with primary distal renal tubular acidosis: a case report. BMC Nephrol. 2018;19:364 (1-6).
33. Liu J, Shen Q, Zhai Y, Fang X, Xu H. Clinical and genetic analysis of distal renal tubular acidosis in three Chinese children. Ren Fail. 2018;40:520–6.
34. Pereira PC, Melo FM, De Marco LA, Oliveira EA, Miranda DM, Silva SE, AC. Whole-exome sequencing as a diagnostic tool for distal renal tubular acidosis. J Pediatr. 2015;91:581–9.
35. Escobar LI, Simian C, TreardC HD, Salvador C, Guerra G, Matos M, Medeiros M, Enciso S, Camargo MD, Vargas-Poussou R. Mutations in *ATP6V1B1 and ATP6V0A4* cause recessive distal renal tubular acidosis in Mexican families. Mol Genet Genomic Med. 2016;4:303–11.
36. Park E, Cho MH, Hyun HS, Shin JI, Lee JH, Park YS, Choi HJ, Kang HG, Cheong HI. Kidney Blood Press Res. 2018;43:513–21.
37. Sharifian M, Esfandiar N, Mazaheri S, Kariminejad A, Mohkam M, Dalirani R, Esmaili R, Ahmadi M, Hassas-Yeganeh M. Distal renal tubular acidosis and its relationship with hearing loss in children: a preliminary report. Iran J Kidney Dis. 2010;4:202–6.
38. Mohebbi N, Vargas-Poussou R, Hegemann SC, Schuknecht B, Kistler AD, Wüthrich RP, Wagner CA. Homozygous and compound heterozygous mutations in the ATP6V1B1 gene in patients with renal tubular acidosis and sensorineural hearing loss. Clin Genet. 2013;83:274–8.
39. Naveen PS, Srikanth L, Venkatesh K, Sarma PV, Sridhar N, Krishnakishore C, Sandeep Y, Manjusha Y, Sivakumar V. Distal renal tubular acidosis with nerve deafness secondary to ATP6B1 gene mutation. Saudi J Kidney Dis Transpl. 2015;26:119–21.
40. Muñoz-Arizpe R, Escobar L, Medeiros M. Sobre-diagnóstico de acidosis tubular renal en México. Rev Investig Clin. 2012;64:399–401.
41. Enerbäck S, Nilsson D, Edwards N, Heglind M, Alkanderi S, Ashton E, Deeb A, Kokash FEB, Bakhsh ARA, Van't Hoff W, Walsh SB, D'Arco F, Daryadel A, Bourgeois S, Wagner CA, Kleta R, Bockenhauer D, Sayer JA. Acidosis and deafness in patients with recessive mutations in FOXI1. J Am Soc Nephrol. 2018;29:1041–8.
42. Vidarsson H, Westergren R, Heglind M, Blomqvist SR, Breton S, Enerbäck S. The forkhead transcription factor Foxi1 is a master regulator of vacuolar H-ATPase proton pumo subunits in the inner ear, kidney and epididymis. PLoS One. 2009;4:e4471.
43. Yenchitsomanus PT, Vasuvattakul S, Kirdpon S, y col. Autosomal recessive distal renal tubular acidosis caused by G701D mutation of anion exchanger 1 gene. Am J Kidney Dis. 2001;40:21–9.
44. Khositseth S, Bruce LJ, Walsh SB, Bawazir WM, Ogle GD, Unwin RJ, Thong MK, Sinha R, Choo KE, Chartapisak W, Kingwatanakul P, Sumboonnanonda A, Vasuvattakul S, Yenchitsomanus P, Wrong O. Tropical distal renal tubular acidosis: clinical and epidemiological studies in 78 patients. QJM. 2012;105:861–77.
45. Alper SL. Familial renal tubular acidosis. J Nephrol. 2010;1:S57–76.
46. Wang D, Yu Y, Wang R, Cai Y, Li Y, Choe CM, Guan H, Wang X. A family with autosomal dominant distal renal tubular acidosis presents with atypical phenotype caused by a Missence mutation (R388C) of the human kidney anion exchanger. Nephron. 2019;141:207–12.
47. Zhang Z, Liu KX, He JW, Fu WZ, Yue H, Zhang H, Zhang CQ, Zhang ZL. Identification of two novel mutations in the SLC4A1 gene in two unrelated Chinese families with distal renal tubular acidosis. Arch Med Res. 2012;43:298–30.

48. Anacleto FE, Bruce LJ, Clayton P, Hegde S, Resontoc LP, Wrong O. Distal renal tubular acidosis in Filipino children, caused by mutations of the anion-exchanger SLC4A1 (AE1, Band 3) gene. Nephron Physiol. 2010;114:19–24.
49. Fry AC, Su Y, Yiu V. col Mutation conferring apical targeting motif on AE1 exchanger causes autosomal dominant distal RTA. J Soc Nephrol. 2012;23:1238–49.
50. Katsura KA, Horst JA, Chandra D, Le TQ, Nakano Y, Zhang Y, Horst OV, Zhu L, Le MH, DenBesten PK. WDR72 models of structure and function: a stage-specific regulator of enamel mineralization. Matrix Biol. 2014;38:48–58.
51. Rungroj N, Nettuwakul C, Sawasdee N, Sangnual S, Deejai N, Misgar RA, Pasena A, Khositseth S, Kirdpon S, Sritippayawan S, Vasuvattakul S, Yenchitsomanus PT. Distal renal tubular acidosis caused by tryptophan-aspartate repeat domain 72 (WDR72) mutations. Clin Genet. 2018;94:409–18.
52. Batlle D, Haque SK. Genetic causes and mechanisms of distal renal tubular acidosis. Nephrol Dial Transplant. 2012;27:3691–704.
53. Sly WS, Whyte MP, Sundaram V, Tashian RE, Hewett-Emmett D, Guibaud P, Vainsel M, Baluarte HJ, Gruskin A, Al-Mosawi M, et al. Carbonic anhydrase II deficiency in 12 families with the autosomal recessive syndrome of osteopetrosis with renal tubular acidosis and cerebral calcification. N Engl J Med. 1985;313:139–45.
54. Fathallah DM, Bejaoui M, Sly WS, Lakhoua R, Dellagi K. A unique mutation underlying carbonic anhydrase II deficiency síndrome in patients of Arab descent. Hum Genet. 1994;94:581–2.
55. Lotan D, Eisenkraft A, Jacobsson JM. Clinical and molecular findings in a family with the carbonic anhydrase II deficiency syndrome. Pediatr Nephrol. 2006;21:423–6.

Chapter 5
History of Renal Tubular Acidosis

Víctor M. García Nieto, Teresa Moraleda Mesa, and Margarita Monge Zamorano

Distal Renal Tubular Acidosis

In 1936, Butler, Wilson, and Farbes published the clinical and biochemical characteristics of four infants between the ages of 2 weeks and 11 months who suffered from a clinical syndrome that had not been described until then, and was characterized by:

(a) Persistent dehydration in the absence of vomiting and excessive diarrhea, in the presence of an adequate intake of food, liquids, and salt.
(b) Persistent hyperpnea associated with a sustained elevation in serum chloride concentration and a reduction in bicarbonate concentration.
(c) Deposit of calcium salts within and adjacent to some renal tubules" [1].

Bicarbonatemia levels ranged from 6 to 12 mEq/l and chloremia levels from 121 to 140 mEq/l. All four children died. In the *post-mortem* study, no pathological evidence of parathyroid hyperplasia was found, which was one of the best-known etiologies of renal calcification of the disease at that time. Another recognized etiology of the same disease was hypervitaminosis D [2]. In the 1930s, some cases had also been described in which calcification of the renal tubules, dehydration, and hypochloremic alkalosis associated with an upper-intestinal obstruction coexisted [1]. With current terminology, we may say that they were cases of chloride deficit or Pseudo-Bartter's syndrome.

In the 1930s, some cases of infants with metabolic acidosis, dehydration, and hypotonia had been published [3], and others more likely with acidosis and

V. M. García Nieto (✉) · M. M. Zamorano
Pediatric Nephrology Section of the University Hospital Nuestra Señora de Candelaria, Santa Cruz de Tenerife, Canary Islands, Spain

T. M. Mesa
Canary Islands, Spain

R. Muñoz (ed.), *Renal Tubular Acidosis in Children*,
https://doi.org/10.1007/978-3-030-91940-5_5

nephrocalcinosis are difficult to guess whether or not they were patients with the same disease [4]. From these cases of nephrocalcinosis in infants, the term "nephrocalcinosis *infantum*" was coined.

In 1940, Albright et al. published the characteristics of a patient that had coincidences with those reported by Butler et al. A 13-year-old girl had persistent rickets and short stature. Plasma calcium levels were normal (ruling out hyperparathyroidism), phosphate levels were reduced, and alkaline phosphatase levels were elevated (consistent with rickets). These symptoms were accompanied by "massive calcium deposits"in the pyramids of the kidneys (Fig. 5.1). Hyperchloremia and low bicarbonate concentration were documented [5]. Stimulating tests were performed using ammonium chloride, sodium citrate, and ammonium nitrate. For the first time in history, the authors concluded that the disease was characterized by an inability to produce ammonia and to excrete acid urine. Likewise, Albright et al. were the first ones to describe the presence of hypercalciuria, which would facilitate the appearance of secondary hyperparathyroidism and, therefore, hypophosphatemia. These authors advocated citrate treatment as a method to "raise serum CO_2 and reduce chloride levels" [5]. Figures 5.2 and 5.3 show the x-rays of both femurs, taken before and after 6 months of treatment. The authors hypothesized that nephrocalcinosis could be the cause of the ammonium secretion defect, an idea that was modified a few years later, by themselves.

Indeed, in 1946, Albright et al., in one of the most extensive articles in Nephrology literature (consisting of 81 pages), believed that nephrocalcinosis should be considered a complication of homeostasis disorders that occur in the new disorder and, named it "renal acidosis resulting from tubular insufficiency without glomerular insufficiency" [6]. The explanation for nephrocalcinosis as a complication seemed obvious since the authors had observed that hypercalciuria was secondary and, normalized once treatment with alkaline salts started. The authors also drew attention to the existence of a urinary loss of potassium that could cause hypokalemia,

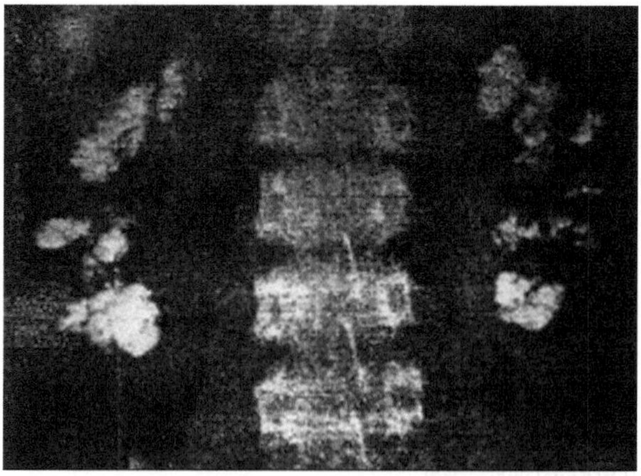

Fig. 5.1 "Dense calcium deposits in the pyramids of both kidneys" on an abdominal radiograph performed in a case of "nephrocalcinosis with rickets, with growth retardation" [5]

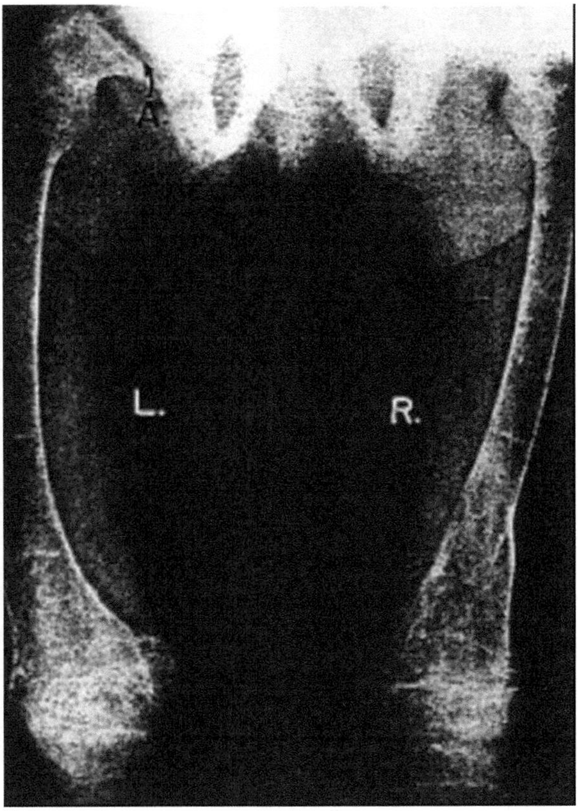

Fig. 5.2 Radiograph of both femurs before starting treatment in the patient in Fig. 5.1 [5]

leading to paralysis. Two patients without renal calcifications showed a more or less acceptable concentration capacity, arguing that hypostenuria should be secondary to nephrocalcinosis.

In the late 1940s, infantile nephrocalcinosis was already related to the presence of hyperchloremic acidosis [7–9]. The disease was also known by the name of Butler-Albright syndrome [10–12], which was combined with that of renal tubular acidosis (RTA) since the early 1950s [13, 14].

In the mid-1950s, family cases began to be published suggesting an autosomal dominant inheritance in some cases of RTA [15–17]. The association between deafness and autosomal recessive inheritance was later described [18–22].

In 1962, a French group [23] and another English group [24] gave an important piece of information describing biochemical data specific to RTA. This was hypocitraturia, which nowadays is an adequate marker of metabolic acidosis. This finding was confirmed soon after [25].

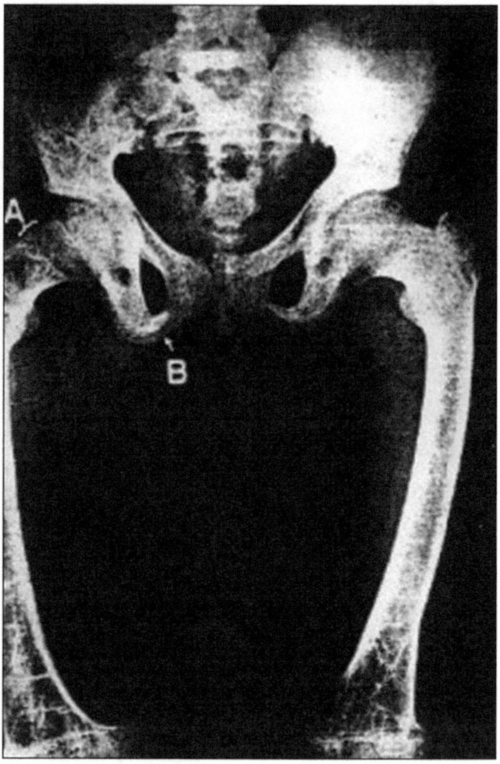

Fig. 5.3 X-ray of the pelvis and both femurs after 6 months of treatment in the same patient in Figs. 5.1 and 5.2 [5]. "An increase in bone density and thickness is observed". "A periosteal new bone border is observed, with remarkable improvement in B"

Transient Tubular Acidosis

In 1953, Lightwood, Payne, and Black described a group of infants diagnosed with a transient variant of RTA. The suppression of alkaline therapy at 2 years of age was not followed by the recurrence of acidosis [26]. This disorder was frequently observed in Great Britain in the 1940s and early 1950s of the last century. However, its frequency decreased dramatically in subsequent years [27], suggesting a causal association with environmental factors such as mercury poisoning [28, 29] or hypercalcemia [30–32]. The excessive addition of vitamin D to milk formulas, a common practice in those years in Great Britain [27], is a theory that could not be neglected regarding the etiology. Likewise, the first sulfamide drugs used could be toxigenic, since years later were known to cause a defect in the renal acidification capacity [33, 34].

The pathophysiology of acidosis in these cases could not be defined, since, in most of them, precise functional studies were not performed, so, given the general knowledge of the time, the syndrome was accepted as the representation of a maturational defect of renal acidification capacity. Currently, some cases of transient distal RTA secondary to poisoning by organophosphate compounds [35] or by viper bite [36] have continued to be published.

As such, the so-called Lightwood syndrome was recognized in the medical literature as a form of transient distal RTA, characteristic of early childhood. The cases of primary proximal RTA described for the first time by Rodríguez-Soriano et al. in 1967 [37] corresponded to a transitory variety [38]. In the chapter written by Drs. Rodríguez Soriano y Vallo in the book published in tribute to Dr. Gustavo Gordillo in 1976, these authors wrote that "the so-called Lightwood syndrome, or transient RTA of the infant, should not be considered as such, since it probably includes various nosological varieties today well recognized" [39].

Transient distal RTA of primary or idiopathic origin was not documented until the mid-1970s. Leumann and Steinmann described the findings in a four-month-old patient with primary distal RTA and loss of bicarbonate. The acidosis did not reappear when the alkaline therapy was suspended, at about 10 months of age, at which time it showed normal tubular function. This patient had transient hypercalcemia, not attributable to vitamin D intoxication or hyperparathyroidism [40]. A similar patient was described at the same time by Hirschman et al. [41]. Likewise, transient "idiopathic" cases of type 4 RTA and hyperkalemia have been described [42, 43]. Other transient cases of type 4 RTA were described due to resistance to aldosterone (obstructive uropathy) [44, 45] or due to an important distal reduction of sodium delivery to the cortical duct, like in patients with nephrotic syndrome, acute diarrhea, etc. [46, 47].

Proximal Tubular Acidosis (PRTA)

Juan Rodríguez Soriano (1933–2010) was an eminent Spanish pediatric nephrologist, educator of several generations of pediatricians, and pediatric nephrologists. He was internationally considered as one of the pioneers of pediatric nephrology and, a benchmark, in that of tubulopathies. His prestige in that specialty was unanimously recognized. He studied Medicine at the University of Barcelona. In 1959, he obtained a scholarship to expand his training at the Hôpital des Enfants Malades in Paris with Pierre Royer and Renée Habib. In 1963 he was admitted to the Albert Einstein College of Medicine in New York. Studies leading to the study of renal acidification capacity under normal circumstances served to identify proximal RTA as an independent pathophysiological entity, a finding that marked his professional life. The work was published in 1967 in *Pediatric Research* [37]. Until then, only distal type 1 RTA was known, which had been described in 1936 by Butler et al. [1], and confirmed 4 years later by Albright et al. [5]. In a subsequent publication by the New York Group, it was learned that patients diagnosed with isolated proximal RTA had had a transient clinical condition [38]. Much later, Dr. Rodríguez Soriano wrote he suspected that PRTA he previously described should have been an immaturity of the Na^+/H^+ (NHE-3) luminal exchanger [48]. In 1970, he took over the Pediatrics Department of the Cruces University Hospital, nearby Bilbao. There, together with Alfredo Vallo, he continued researching and publishing on many pediatric topics,

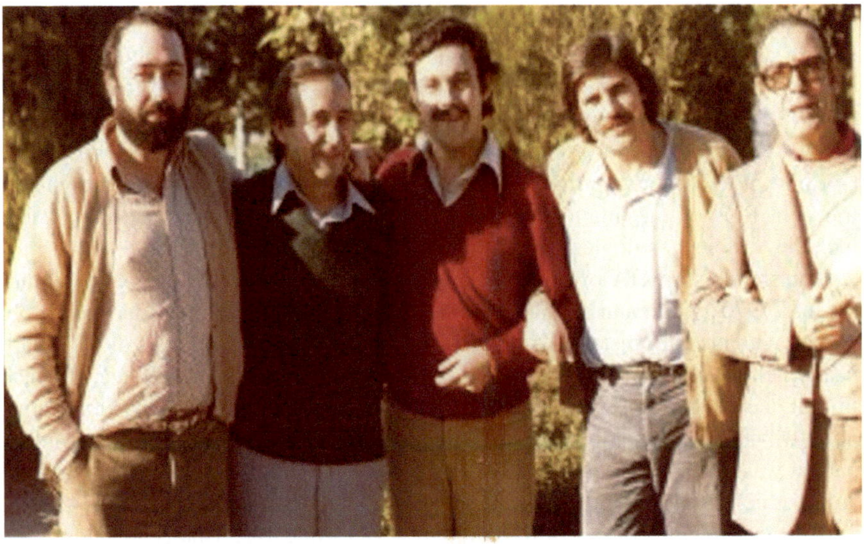

Fig. 5.4 The Bilbao Pediatric Nephrology Group after the VI National Meeting of Pediatric Nephrology (Granada, November 1978). From left to right, Gonzalo Castillo (†), Alfredo Vallo (†), Víctor M. García Nieto, Roberto Oliveros and Juan Rodríguez Soriano (†). This image is the property of one of the authors (VMGN)

but especially on various aspects of his two main topics of interest, kidney function tests and tubulopathies [49] (Fig. 5.4).

Since his stay in Paris, he had been interested in distal ATR [50] and continued to be a priority object of study for the Group formed in Bilbao. Thus, in 1975 they demonstrated, through low-saline fluid overload, that in infants with distal RTA, there could be an associated urinary loss of sodium and bicarbonate, motivated by an increase in the distal supply of both ions [51].

At the V National Meeting of Pediatric Nephrology (Madrid, 1977), the Group presented the results obtained with the stimulating test to increase secretion of hydrogen ions in alkaline urine by measuring urinary pCO_2, both in normal children and children with kidney problems [52]. In the early 1980s, they published several laboratory tests, corroborating that some patients who did not increase urinary after a fluid load with a high bicarbonate concentration could increase urinary pCO_2 after the administration of phosphate, thus suggesting that this renal tubular response could be applied in the evaluation and understanding of the etiology of renal tubular acidosis [53].

In 1981, Rodriguez Soriano et al. published the long-term evolution of five patients with distal RTA. The authors stated that with adequate treatment, they all had normal glomerular filtration rate, optimal growth and development, a halt in the progression of nephrocalcinosis, and the absence of another clinical data characteristic of the disease, except for persistent polyuria [54].

The Other Forms of Renal Tubular Acidosis

In 1972, two independent groups published the first cases of type 3 RTA associated with osteopetrosis. Sly et al. described three sisters with a form of osteopetrosis different from the varieties known until then, namely the malignant type and the benign autosomal dominant type. Patients with this disorder showed clinical manifestations by the age of 2 years, mainly bone fractures. Other signs were short stature, mental retardation, mild anemia, dental malocclusion, and visual impairment due to compression of the optic nerve [55].

The same year, Guibaud et al. described two brothers with renal tubular acidosis and mild osteopetrosis, both unaffected parents, originally from North Africa, were first cousins [56]. In 1983, Sly et al. demonstrated the absence of type II carbonic anhydrase in red blood cells of affected patients [57]. Confirmation of this deficit using molecular biology techniques was carried out by Venta et al. in 1991 [58].

The first patients with type 4 RTA and hyperkalemia were cases secondary to Gordon's syndrome [59, 60], hypoaldosteronism [61], and obstructive uropathy [44].

References

1. Butler AM, Wilson JL, Farber S. Dehydration and acidosis with calcification at renal tubules. J Pediatr. 1936;8:489–99.
2. Thatcher L. Hypervitaminosis-D with report of a fatal case in a child. Edinburgh Med. 1931;38:457–67.
3. Lightwood R, MacLagan NF, Williams JG. Persistent acidosis in an infant: cause not yet ascertained. Proc R Soc Med. 1936;29:1431–3.
4. Lightwood R. Calcium infarction of the kidneys in infants. Arch Dis Child. 1935;10:205–6.
5. Albright F, Consolazio WV, Coombs FS, Sulkowitch HW, Talbott JH. Metabolic studies and therapy in a case of nephrocalcinosis with rickets and dwarfism. Bull Johns Hopk Hosp. 1940;66:7–33.
6. Albright F, Burnett CH, Parson W, Reifenstein EC, Roos A. Osteomalacia and late rickets. The various etiologies met in the United States with emphasis on that resulting from a specific form of renal acidosis, the therapeutic indications for each etiological sub-group, and the relationship between osteomalacia and Milkman's syndrome. Medicine (Baltimore). 1946;25:399–479.
7. Boutourline-Young HJ. Nephrocalcinosis infantum with hyperchloraemic acidosis. Br Med J. 1949;1:181–3.
8. Latner AL, Burnard EC. Idiopathic hyperchloraemic renal acidosis of infants (*nephrocalcinosis infantum*). Observations on the site and nature of the lesion. Q J Med. 1950;19:285–301.
9. Farrell RH. Hyperchloraemic renal acidosis of infants (*nephrocalcinosis infantum*); report of a case and review of literature. Guys Hosp Rep. 1953;102:234–9.
10. Faber HK, Abramson M, Silverberg RJ. The Butler-Albright syndrome of tubular nephropathy; acidosis, late rickets, dwarfing, diabetes insipidus, and nephrocalcinosis. Stanford Med Bull. 1948;6:157–74.
11. Legrain M. Primary hyperchloremic acidosis (Lightwood-Butler-Albright syndrome). Gaz Med Fr. 1957;64:1749–50.

12. Schmuziger P, Pfisterer R, Baechtold H, Truniger B. Renal tubular hyperchloremic acidosis (Lightwood-Butler-Albright syndrome). Schweiz Med Wochenschr. 1961;91:506–15.
13. Pines KL, Mudge GH. Renal tubular acidosis with osteomalacia; report of 3 cases. Am J Med. 1951;11:302–11.
14. Foss GL, Perry CB, Wood FJ. Renal tubular acidosis. Q J Med. 1956;25:185–99.
15. Pitts HH Jr, Schulte JW, Smith DR. Nephrocalcinosis in a father and three children. J Urol. 1955;73:208–11.
16. Huth EJ, Webster GD Jr, Elkinton JR. The renal excretion of hydrogen ion in renal tubular acidosis: III. An attempt to detect latent cases in a family; comments on nosology, genetics and etiology of the primary disease. Am J Med. 1960;29:586–98.
17. Richards P, Wrong OM. Dominant inheritance in a family with familial renal tubular acidosis. Lancet. 1972;2:998–9.
18. Royer P, Broyer M. L'acidoserenale au cours des tubulopathies congénitales. In: Proceedings of ActualitésNephrologiques de l'Hopital Necker. Paris: Flammarion; 1967. p. 73.
19. Nance WE, Sweeney A. Evidence for autosomal recessive inheritance of the syndrome of renal tubular acidosis with deafness. Birth Defects Orig Artic Ser. 1971;7:70–2.
20. Walker WG. Renal tubular acidosis and deafness. Birth Defects Orig Artic Ser. 1971;7:126.
21. Cohen T, Brand-Auraban A, Karshai C, Jacob A, Gay I, Tsitsianov J, et al. Familial infantile renal tubular acidosis and congenital nerve deafness: an autosomal recessive syndrome. Clin Genet. 1973;4:275–8.
22. Dunger DB, Brenton DP, Cain AR. Renal tubular acidosis and nerve deafness. Arch Dis Child. 1980;55:221–5.
23. Royer P, Lestradet H, Nordmann R, Mathieu H, Rodríguez-Soriano J. Études sur quatre cas d'ac idosetubulairechroniqueidiopathiqueavechypocitraturie. Ann Pediatr (Paris). 1962;38:808–29.
24. Dedmon RE, Wrong O. The excretion of organic anion in renal tubular acidosis with particular reference to citrate. Clin Sci. 1962;22:19–32.
25. Nordin BE, Smith DA. Citric acid excretion in renal stone disease and in renal tubular acidosis. Br J Urol. 1963;35:438–44.
26. Lightwood R, Payne WW, Black JA. Infantile renal acidosis. Pediatrics. 1953;12:628–44.
27. Lightwood R, Butler N. Decline in primary infantile renal acidosis: aetiological implications. Br Med J. 1963;1:855–7.
28. MacGregor ME, Rayner PH. Pink disease and primary renal tubular acidosis. A common cause. Lancet. 1964;2:1083–5.
29. Simister JM. Pink disease and primary renal tubular acidosis. Lancet. 1964;2:1296.
30. Doxiadis SA. Idiopathic renal acidosis in infancy. Arch Dis Child. 1952;27:409–27.
31. Carre IJ, Wood BS, Smallwood WC. Idiopathic renal acidosis in infancy. Arch Dis Child. 1954;29:326–33.
32. Galán E. Acidosis hiperclorémica renal (síndrome de Butler-Lightwood-Albright) provocada por hipervitaminosis D y efecto curativo de la ACTH. Rev Cubana Pediatr. 1955;27:199–218.
33. Murphy JL, Griswold WR, Reznik VM, Mendoza SA. Trimethoprim/sulfamethoxazole-induced renal tubular acidosis. Child Nephrol Urol. 1990;10:49–50.
34. Lin SH, Kuo AA, Yu FC, Lin YF. Reversible voltage-dependent distal renal tubular acidosis in a patient receiving standard doses of trimethoprim-sulphamethoxazole. Nephrol Dial Transplant. 1997;12:1031–3.
35. Narayan R, Abdulla MC, Alungal J. Transient distal renal tubular acidosis in organophosphate poisoning. Indian J Crit Care Med. 2017;21:170–1.
36. Weerakkody RM, Lokuliyana PN, Lanerolle RD. Transient distal renal tubular acidosis following hump nosed viper bite: two cases from Sri Lanka. Saudi J Kidney Dis Transpl. 2016;27:1018–20.
37. Rodríguez Soriano J, Boichis H, Stark H, Edelmann CM Jr. Proximal renal tubular acidosis. A defect in bicarbonate reabsorption with normal urinary acidification. Pediatr Res. 1967;1:81–98.
38. Nash MA, Torrado AD, Greifer I, Spitzer A, Edelmann CM Jr. Renal tubular acidosis in infants and children. J Pediatr. 1972;80:738–48.

39. Rodríguez Soriano J, Vallo A. Acidosis tubular renal en el lactante. Actualización del síndrome de Lightwood. Mota F, editor. En: Tópicos Selectos de Nefrología. México DF: Nueva Ed. Interamericana; 1976, pp. 333–346.
40. Leumann EP, Steinmann B. Persistent and transient distal renal tubular acidosis with bicarbonate wasting. Pediatr Res. 1975;9:767–73.
41. Hirschman GH, Beale MG, Rao DD, Ellis D, Chan JCM. Transientprimary distal renal tubular acidosis. Kidney Int. 1975;8:413.
42. Donckerwolcke RA, Valk C, van Wijngaarden-Penterman MJG, van Stekelenburg GJ. A case of transient renal tubular acidosis type 1,4 hybrid RTA: a study of the pathophysiologic characteristics of the acidification defect. Pediatr Res. 1979;13:1177–8.
43. Khositseth S. Transient hyperkalemic distal renal tubular acidosis with bicarbonate wasting in a young child. J Med Assoc Thail. 2011;94(Suppl 7):S204–7.
44. Batlle DC, Arruda JA, Kurtzman NA. Hyperkalemic distal renal tubular acidosis associated with obstructive uropathy. N Engl J Med. 1981;304:373–80.
45. Rodríguez-Soriano J, Vallo A, Oliveros R, Castillo G. Transient pseudohypoaldosteronism secondary to obstructive uropathy in infancy. J Pediatr. 1983;103:375–80.
46. Rodriguez-Soriano J, Vallo A, Castillo G, Oliveros R. Defect in urinary acidification in nephrotic syndrome and its correction by furosemide. Nephron. 1982;32:308–13.
47. Izraeli S, Rachmel A, Frishberg Y, Erman A, Flasterstein B, Nitzan M, at al. Transient renal acidification defect during acute infantile diarrhea: the role of urinary sodium. J Pediatr. 1990;117:711–6.
48. Rodríguez-Soriano J. New insights into the pathogenesis ofrenal tubular acidosis –from functional to molecular studies. Pediatr Nephrol. 2000;14:1121–36.
49. García Nieto VM, Grünberg J, Luis Yanes MI. Discípulos y maestros. Lo que aprendimos de Juan Rodríguez Soriano. Rev Esp Pediatr. 2011;67:324–31.
50. Royer P, Lestradet H, Rodríguez-Soriano J. Acidosis tubular crónica idiopática en la infancia. Exploraciones funcionales en tres observaciones. Rev Esp Pediatr. 1961;17:661–83.
51. Rodríguez-Soriano J, Vallo A, Garcia-Fuentes M. Distal renaltubular acidosis in infancy: a bicarbonatewastingstate. J Pediatr. 1975;86:524–32.
52. Quintela MJ, Vallo A, Oliveros R, et al. Determinación de la $pC0_2$ urinaria en el estudio de la capacidad de acidificación distal. AnEsp Pediatr. 1978;11:443–4.
53. Vallo A, Rodríguez-Soriano J. Oral phosphate-loading test for the assessment of distal urinary acidification in children. Miner Electrolyte Metab. 1984;10:387–90.
54. Rodríguez-Soriano J, Vallo A, Castillo G, Oliveros R. Natural history of primary distal renal tubular acidosis treated since infancy. J Pediatr. 1982;101:669–76.
55. Sly WS, Lang R, Avioli L, Haddad J, Lubowitz H, McAlister W. Recessive osteopetrosis: new clinical phenotype. Am J Hum Genet. 1972;24:34A.
56. Guibaud P, Larbre F, Freycon MT, Genoud J. Osteopetrose et acidoserenaletubulaire. Deux cas de cette association dans unefratrie. Arch Franc Pediatr. 1972;29:269–86.
57. Sly WS, Hewett-Emmett D, Whyte MP, Yu YS, Tashian RE. Carbonic anhydrase II deficiency identified as the primary defect in the autosomal recessive syndrome of osteopetrosis with renal tubular acidosis and cerebral calcification. Proc Natl Acad Sci U S A. 1983;80:2752–6.
58. Venta PJ, Welty RJ, Johnson TM, Sly WS, Tashian RE. Carbonic anhydrase II deficiency syndrome in a Belgian family is caused by a point mutation at an invariant histidine residue (107 His----Tyr): complete structure of the normal human CA II gene. Am J Hum Genet. 1991;49:1082–90.
59. Arnold JE, Healy JK. Hyperkalemia, hypertension and systemic acidosis without renal failure associated with a tubular defect in potassium excretion. Am J Med. 1969;47:461–72.
60. Spitzer A, Edelmann CM Jr, Goldberg LD, Henneman PH. Short stature, hyperkalemia and acidosis: a defect in renal transport of potassium. Kidney Int. 1973;3:251–7.
61. Hulter HN, Licht JH, Glynn RD, Sebastian A. Renal acidosis in mineralocorticoid deficiency is not dependent on NaCl depletion or hyperkalemia. Am J Phys. 1979;236:F283–94.

Chapter 6
Classification of Renal Tubular Acidosis

Norma Elizabeth Guerra Hernández

Renal tubular acidosis (RTA) is characterized biochemically by persistent metabolic acidosis, hyperchloremia, and a normal anion gap. Table 6.1 shows the classification of RTAs into 4 types, which may be distinguished from each other based on the clinical findings, pathophysiological mechanisms, specific molecular changes that generate the RTA, and the results of the different diagnostic tests [1].

Recent advances in molecular biology techniques allow us to understand the pathophysiological mechanisms and the defect of the different transporters that

Table 6.1 Classification of renal tubular acidosis

Type	Name	Tubular area affected	Main defect
Type 1	Distal or classic RTA	Collecting duct α-intercalated cell	Inability to secrete H^+ ions and ammonium H^+-ATP-ase, AE1
Type 2	Proximal RTA	Proximal tubule	Bicarbonate reabsorption (HCO_3^-) NBCe1 exchanger
Type 3	Mixed distal and proximal RTA	Combined proximal tubule and distal collecting tubule	H^+ excretion and HCO_3^- reabsorption (osteopetrosis, brain calcifications)
Type 4	Distal RTA with hyperkalemia	Collecting tubule	Pseudohypoaldosteronismo or hypoaldesteronismo (ENaC, Na^+K^+ATPase, NCC)

N. E. G. Hernández (✉)
Department of Pediatric Nephrology, General "Dr. Gaudencio González Garza," National Medical Center La Raza, Mexican Institute of Social Security, Mexico City, Mexico

Advanced Studies Iztacalaca Faculty, National Autonomous University of Mexico, Mexico City, Mexico

R. Muñoz (ed.), *Renal Tubular Acidosis in Children*,
https://doi.org/10.1007/978-3-030-91940-5_6

Table 6.2 Hereditary characteristics of primary RTA

	Inheritance	Chromosome	Gen mutation	Defect
Proximal RTA (type 2)				
Autosomal dominant	AD	?	?	?
Autosomal recessive with ocular abnormalities	AR	4q21	SLC4A4	Cotransporter NBCe1
Sporadic in lactating babies	AR	–	–	NHE3 antiporter immaturity?
Distal RTA (type 1)				
Autosomal dominant	AD	17q21-22	SLC4A1	AE1
Autosomal recessive with early deafness	AR	2p13	ATP6V1B1	B1 subunit of H^+-ATPase
Autosomal recessive with or without early deafness	AR	7q33-34	ATP6V0A4	A4 subunit of H^+-ATPase
Mixed RTA (type 3)				
Autosomal recessive with osteopetrosis	AR	8q22	CA II	Carbonic anhydrase type II (CA II)
ATR Hyperkalemic (type 4)				
Pseudohypoaldosteronism type 1				
Autosomal dominant (renal)	AD	4q31.1	MR	Mineralocorticoid receptor (MR)
Autosomal recessive	AR	16p12	SNCC1B, SCNN1G	β and γ ENaC (sodium epithelial channel)
Pseudohypoaldosteronism type 2 (Gordon's syndrome)	AD	12p13.3 17p11-q21	WNK1 WNK4	WNK1 kinase WNK4 kinase

participate in the regulation of the acid-base balance, allowing a better understanding of the different forms of presentation and hereditary syndromes [1, 2].

Each of the different types of RTA may present in the hereditary or primary form or acquired, a secondary form [2]. The primary forms are the result of the genetic defect in the transporters or enzymes involved in the reabsorption of HCO_3^- or the secretion of H^+ and ammonium ions; it is more frequent in childhood (Table 6.2) [1–4]. Secondary forms usually occur in adults and are the result of exposure to drugs or toxins, or secondary to systemic or immunological diseases [1, 2].

Proximal Renal Tubular Acidosis (Type 2)

It is characterized by a defect in proximal tubular reabsorption of HCO_3^-. It may be an isolated alteration, unrelated to other tubular abnormalities, or more frequently accompanied by other tubular defects, such as glycosuria, hyperuricosuria, hyperphosphaturia, and aminoaciduria, causing Toni-Debré-Fanconi syndrome, secondary to cystinosis, and Lowe's syndrome, among other causes [5, 6].

They can also occur in hereditary form or secondary to the administration of medications or be associated with different diseases. The main manifestations are failure to thrive, vomiting, anorexia, rickets, and osteoporosis: In severe cases, ocular malformations and mental retardation are also observed [2, 5, 6].

Distal Renal Tubular Acidosis (Type 1)

This type of RTA is characterized by the inability of the α-intercalated cells of the collecting tubule to secrete hydrogen (H^+). The clinical presentation usually begins within the first year of life, with persistent metabolic acidosis, normal anion gap, hypercalciuria, hypocitraturia, and nephrocalcinosis, which may be evident in the first weeks of life, and is frequently associated with early or late sensorineural deafness [1, 2, 4, 6, 7].

Five genetic mutations are the etiology of RTAd that have been identified in the genetic or primary forms, namely SLC4A1, ATP6V0A4, ATP6V1B1, FOXI1, and WDR72, as appear in Table 6.2 and will be described in greater detail in the corresponding chapter [2, 6, 7].

According to the specific defects in urinary acidification, the distal RTA is classified as:

(a) Secretory defect:

It is characterized by a defect in cellular function that can affect both the luminal H^+-ATPase pump, as well as the action of intracellular type II carbonic anhydrase or the basolateral AE1 anion exchanger (Fig. 6.1).

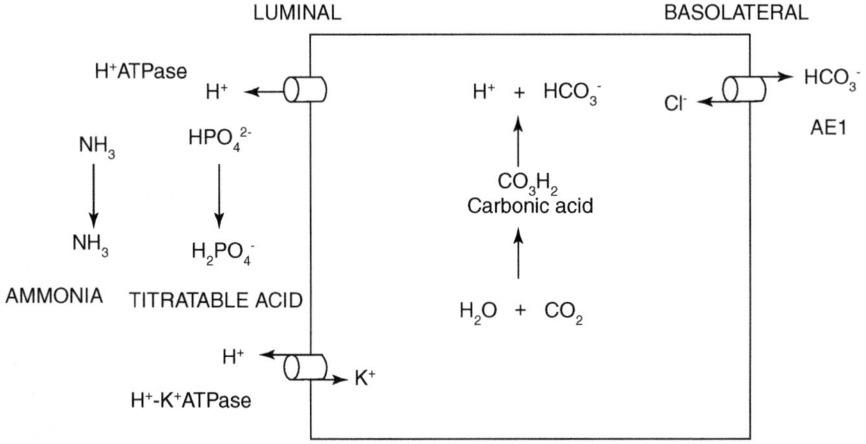

Fig. 6.1 Cortical collecting tubule

(b) Voltage defect (short circuit defect):

Generated by the inability of the distal tubule to increase or generate the intratubular electrical gradient for H^+ ion secretion, together with impaired K^+ secretion. This alteration is due to a defect in the arrival or transport of sodium at that level. It is also associated with hyperkalemia due to diminished potassium secretion, as occurs in type 4 or hyperkalemic RTA. This alteration is observed in children with type 1 primary pseudohypoaldosteronism and is associated with mutations in the epithelial sodium channel-forming subunits (ENaC) [3, 5, 8].

(c) Gradient defect (increased back diffusion):

There is a normal H^+ ion renal secretory capacity. However, excretion is ineffective due to the presence of back diffusion of the secreted H^+ ions, as a consequence of increased permeability in the luminal membrane. This defect occurs in distal renal tubular acidosis secondary to the use of amphotericin B [8].

(d) Hydrogen ion buffering defect:

It is a result of the decrease in phosphate and NH3 (ammonium) buffering capacity. The most frequent etiology of this alteration is the defect in the transport of NH_3 from the proximal nephron to the distal areas, as a consequence of a chronic tubulointerstitial medullary pathology primary or secondary to nephrocalcinosis [8].

(e) H^+ ion unavailability defect:

A feasible explanation may be the presence of a minor secretion of H^+or voltage defects; it has been described in adult patients with prolonged treatment with lithium salts, but also may be seen in inherited forms of distal RTA [3, 5, 8].

Type 3 Renal Tubular Acidosis

Functional characteristics of both forms of ATR, proximal and distal, are shared. There is a defect in the tubular reabsorption of the filtered HCO_3–, but unlike isolated proximal RTA, there is also an inability to acidify the urine [2, 3]. It is characterized by a hereditary deficiency of type II carbonic anhydrase, necessary for proximal and distal renal acidification, as well as for osteoclastic function and brain maturation [6]. It is observed in autosomal recessive osteopetrosis and is secondary to mutations in the CA II gene, which encodes carbonic anhydrase type II, generating RTA with cerebral calcifications and mental retardation [2, 5].

Type 4 Renal Tubular Acidosis

The acid-base imbalance is generated by the deficiency or resistance to aldosterone causing metabolic acidosis with hyperkalemia [1]. It occurs more frequently in adults [3]. It has been identified in patients with pseudohypoaldosteronism and

Table 6.3 Clinical characteristics of RTA

	RTA type 1	RTA type 2	RTA type 3	RTA type 4
During acidosis				
Anion Gap	Normal	Normal	Normal	Normal
Urinary ammonium	Low	Normal	Low	Low
Serum potassium	Low /normal	Low /normal	Low /normal	High
Minimum urinary pH	>5.5	<5.5	>5.5	<5.5
With normal serum bicarbonate				
Fractional excretion of bicarbonate	<5%	>10–15%	>5%	>5–10%
Maximum urinary pCO_2 (mmHg)	<60–70	>60–70	<60–70	>60–70
pCO_2 urine: plasma ratio (mmHg)	<20	>20	<20	>20

primary hypoaldosteronism, congenital adrenal hyperplasia, obstructive uropathy, and nephrotic syndrome, as well as associated with the use of medications, such as trimethoprim, pentamidine, cyclosporine A, and lithium [2, 9]. In this type of RTA, the patients keep the capacity of urinary acidification, achieving a urine pH <5.5 after an acid load, but there is an inability to increase urinary excretion of pCO_2 in clinical situations of systemic metabolic acidosis [4].

According to the laboratory findings, the different types of RTA have specific characteristics that allow differential diagnosis and, therefore, the therapeutic approach, as shown in Table 6.3 [1, 10].

References

1. Gil-Peña H, et al. Renal tubular acidosis. J Pediatr. 2014;164:691–8.
2. Rodriguez-Soriano J. Renal tubular acidosis: the clinical entity. J Am Soc Nephrol. 2002;13:2160–70.
3. García-Nieto VM, Luis-Yanes MI. Acidosis tubular renal, en Anton M y Rodriguez LM, Nefrología Pediátrica, Manual Práctico, Asociaci0n Española de Nefrología Pediátrica (AENP); 2010. pp. 155–163.
4. Aguirre Meñica M, Luis Yanes MI. Tubulopatías. Protoc diagn ter pediatr. 2014;1:135–53.
5. Yaxley J, Pirrone C. Review of the diagnostic evaluation of renal tubular acidosis. Ochsner J. 2016;16:525–30.
6. Finer G, Landau D. Clinical approach to proximal renal tubular acidosis in children. Adv Chronic Kidney Dis. 2018;25:351–7.
7. López-García S. Treatment and long-term outcome in primary distal renal tubular acidosis. Nephrol Dial Transplant. 2019;34:981.
8. Rodríguez Soriano J, Vallo Boado A. Acidosis tubular renal en García Nieto VM, Santos Rodríguez F, Rodriguez Iturbe B, Nefrología Pediátrica, 2006; pp. 207–219.
9. Sharma S. Comprehensive clinical approach to renal tubular acidosis. Clin Exp Nephrol. 2015;19:556–61.
10. Santos F, Ordoñez F. Clinical and laboratory approaches in the diagnosis of renal tubular acidosis. Pediatr Nephrol. 2015;30:2099–107.

Chapter 7
Laboratory Diagnosis of Renal Tubular Acidosis. Acidification Tests

Víctor M. García Nieto, María Isabel Luis Yanes, and Patricia Tejera Carreño

Simple Determinations

Blood

(a) Hyperchloremia. Although it is not a sensu stricto functional test, it should be remembered that from its initial description, it is known that hyperchloremia is a characteristic sign of renal tubular acidosis (RTA) [1]. Hyperchloremia is accompanied by a normal anion gap [2] (Fig. 7.1). However, not all cases of RTA have hyperchloremia [3].
(b) Anion gap. The calculation of the plasma anion gap helps to study the origin of metabolic acidosis.

$$\text{The formula is : pNa}^{+} - \left[\text{Cl}^{-}\right]\text{p} + \left[\text{HCO}_{3}^{-}\right]\text{p}$$

Hyperchloremic RTA presents with a normal anion gap. In contrast, anion gap values rise in various disorders that occur with increased acid production and normochloremia, as in ketoacidosis, lactic acidosis, kidney failure, or salicylate poisoning [4, 5] (Fig. 7.2).

V. M. García Nieto (✉) · M. I. L. Yanes
Pediatric Nephrology Section of the University Hospital Nuestra Señora de Candelaria, Santa Cruz de Tenerife, Canary Islands, Spain

P. T. Carreño
Pediatric Emergency Service, University Hospital, Hospital Universitario Insular Materno Infantil, Las Palmas de Gran Canaria, Canary Islands, Spain

R. Muñoz (ed.), *Renal Tubular Acidosis in Children*,
https://doi.org/10.1007/978-3-030-91940-5_7

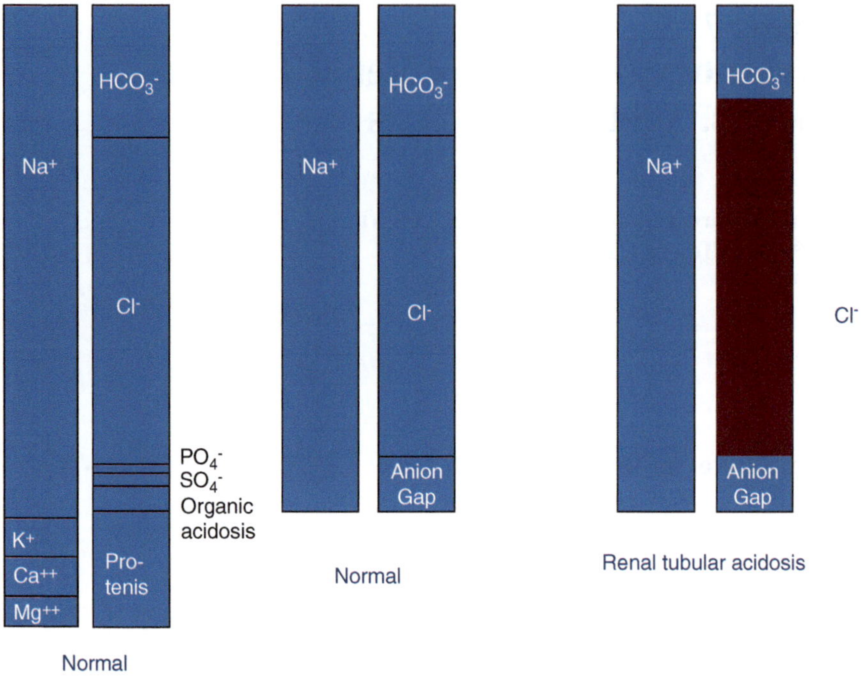

Fig. 7.1 Graphic representation, in the form of a Gamble nomogram, on the composition of the plasma showing the physiological electro neutrality (left) (2), the concept of anion gap (center) and the behavior of chloride levels and anion gap in patients with RTA (right)

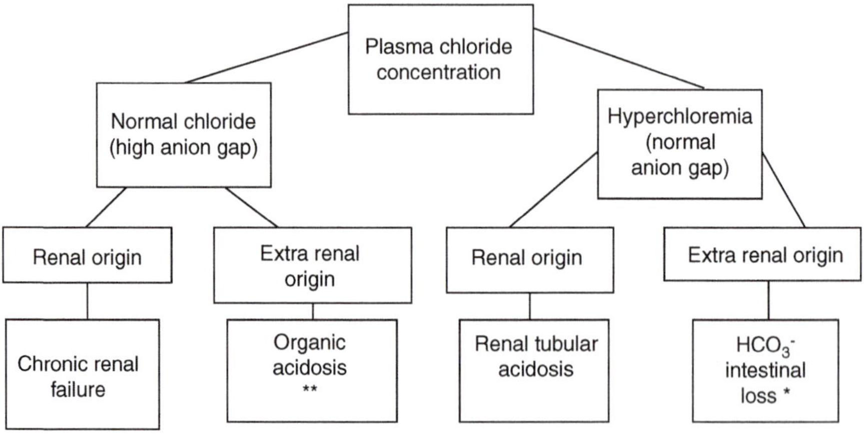

*Diarrhea, ureterosigmoidostomy, pancreatic and, biliary looses, cholestiramine therapy, acute enterocolitis due to cow's milk protein intolerance (lactating age)

**Lactic acidosis, diabetic ketoacidosis, starvation acidosis, ethylene glycol ingestion, methanol, salicylates intoxication

Fig. 7.2 Algorithm on the etiology of metabolic acidosis from plasma chloride levels

The normal value of the anion gap varies according to laboratory techniques and whether or not the K^+ concentration is included in the formula. Thus, values between 3 and 11 mEq/l have been described as normal when "ion selectivity electrodes" are used. If the photometry technique is used to measure the concentration of Na^+ and K^+ and the colorimetric technique to measure the concentration of bicarbonate [HCO_3^-] plus chloride concentration [Cl^-], the normal value is 8–16 mEq/l, but the value increases to 10–20 mEq/l if the concentration of plasma potassium [K^+] is also included in the formula.

Urine

(a) Hypercalciuria and hypocitraturia. The frequency of hypercalciuria and, especially, of hypocitraturia is very high in cases of RTA. Citrate is a very sensitive marker of metabolic acidosis [6]. When the pH of the proximal tubular cell becomes low, the activity of the sodium-dependent dicarboxylate transporter 1 (NADC1) which is located in the apical membrane of the proximal tubule is stimulated. NADC1 is an electrogenic transporter coupled to Na^+ reabsorption at a rate of 3 Na^+ cations for 1 citrate$^{2-/3-}$ anion [2]. The result of increased citrate tubular reabsorption is hypocitraturia. Much of citrate metabolism and its tubular reabsorption depends on the action of citrate-lyase and the mitochondrial-aconitase ATP which transforms citrate into iso-citrate to enter the Krebs cycle [7]. Citrate participates in the Krebs cycle in the mitochondria, thereby producing a greater amount of CO_2 that is transported into the cell cytoplasm. When citrate$^{2-/3-}$ is converted to CO_2 and H_2O three $H^+$are consumed, a reaction equivalent to generating bicarbonate.

During an acid overload, the activity of citrate-lyase and the mitochondrial-aconitase ATP increases concomitantly with a decrease in the concentration of citrate at the renal cortical level [8]. Intracellular hypocitraturia stimulates the entry of more citrate into the cell through the activation of NADC1. In summary, hypocitraturia can be an indicator of metabolic acidosis and RTA.

(b) Anion gap in the urine. Anion gap is an indirect marker of NH_4^+ excretion in the urine. Under normal conditions, the total charge of positive ions that appear in the urine ($UNa^+ + UK^+ + UCa^{2+} + UMg^{2+} + UNH_4^+$) equals the total negative charge of urinary ions (UCl^- + organic Uanions+$UHCO_3^-$ + USO_4^- + $UH_2PO_4^-$/HPO_4^{2-}), such that:

$$UNa^+ + UK^+ + UCa^{2+} + UMg^{2+} + UNH_4^+ = UCl^- + \text{organic Uanions}$$
$$+ UHCO_3^- + USO_4^{2-} + UH_2PO_4^- / HPO_4^{2-}$$

Assuming that the urinary concentrations of cations and anions other than Na^+, K^+, Cl^-, and NH_4^+ do not change significantly after an acid overload (an assumption that is not entirely correct), the initial formula would become:

$$UNa^+ + UK^+ + UNH_4^+ = UCl^-$$

Urinary UNH_4^+ reduction is accompanied by UCl^- reduction to maintain electroneutrality and vice versa. Therefore, the urinary NH_4^+ concentration can be estimated by subtracting the Cl^- concentration from the sum of the Na^+ and K^+ concentrations, according to the following formula [9–11]:

$$UNH_4^+ \left(\text{anion gap}\right) = \left(UNa^+ + UK^+\right) - UCl^-$$

Thus, in a distal RTA, the anion gap is positive [$(UNa^+ + UK^+) > UCl^-$], since less ammonium production goes along with a decreased chloride excretion. On the other hand, when there is intestinal or renal loss (proximal tubular acidosis) of bicarbonate, the urinary anion gap (NH_4^+) is negative [$UCl^- > UNa^+ + UK^+$)]. Calculation of the anion gap can help to differentiate distal from proximal renal tubular acidosis.

Generally speaking, urinary anion gap values range from −20 to −50 mEq/L in individuals who may excrete adequate amounts of NH_4^+ [10, 11]. On the contrary, as indicated, it is less negative or even positive in individuals in whom urinary excretion of NH_4^+ is reduced [11].

Batlle et al. studied seven normal subjects who received an ammonium chloride overload during three days, the urine anion gap was negative (−27 ± 9.8 mmol/l) and the urinary pH was less than 5.3 (4.9 ± 0.03). Also, in eight patients with diarrhea, the urine anion gap was negative (−20 ± 5.7 mmol/l). In contrast, the urinary anion gap was positive in all patients with impaired renal acidification capacity, both in the distal RTA type 1(23 ± 4.1 mmol/l; 11 patients) and in RTA type 4 (hyperkalemic RTA) (30 ± 4.2; 12 patients), as well as in 15 patients with selective aldosterone deficiency (39 ± 4.2) [11].

The urine anion gap should be only calculated in the presence of systemic metabolic acidosis.

Tests in Which H^+ Secretion Is Stimulated by an Acid Overload

Acidification Test with Ammonium Chloride ($ClNH_4$)

This is the traditional test to diagnose distal RTA, to find out if the excretion of hydrogen ions is adequate or not. It was the first test developed for this purpose [12, 13]. The overload of acid radicals provided by $ClNH_4$ stimulates its secretion by the H^+ATPase of the α-intercalated cells of the cortical collecting duct. Acidosis also stimulates the proximal production of ammonia and its delivery to the collecting tubule. Currently, the test is performed less frequently because it is poorly tolerated, with gastritis, nausea, vomiting, and severe metabolic acidosis. The test is altered in patients with distal RTA due to the defect of hydrogen secretion.

After emptying the bladder, 75–100 mEq/m^2 of $ClNH_4$ (1 g = 18.8 mEq) are administered orally, in enteric protection capsules (in adults or adolescents, the dose is 0.1 g/kg) [14]. Urine samples are collected at 60-minute intervals during the following 4–6 hours. Urine volume and urine pH are measured. Titratable acid and ammonia are determined in the two urine specimens with the lowest pH.

In some selected patients, if necessary, the test can be done by intravenous infusion of $ClNH_4$0.9‰ (100 mEq/m^2) for 4–6 hours.

Another way to perform the test is the so-called "long test", in which similar doses of $ClNH_4$ are administered, divided into three doses over three days [14]. This modality is the most accurate to assess the renal capacity to generate ammonium since it takes several days to do so.

A normal response implies a decrease in urine pH < 5.35. The normal values in infants and older children for titratable acid and ammonium excretion in both "short" and "long" tests [14–16].

Tests Performed with Another Source of Hydrogen Production

In addition to ammonium chloride, L-arginine monohydrochloride ($C_6H_{14}N_4O_2$) [17–19] has also been used as a stimulus to acidify the urine.

Tests in Which the Secretion of Hydrogen Ions Is Stimulated by an Increase in Tubular Electronegativity

Acidification Test with Furosemide (Stimulus to Acidify in Acidic Urine)

(a) Classic test. In 1968, Puschett and Goldberg demonstrated that acute administration of furosemide induces the production of acidic urine [20]. Subsequently, other authors demonstrated its utility in the study of renal acidification capacity [21–24].

Furosemide reduces the reabsorption of sodium, potassium, and chloride in the ascending limb of Henle's loop by inhibiting the cotransporter $Na^+K^+2Cl^-$ (NKCC2, Na-K-Cl cotransporter) [25]. The volume contraction generated by the diuretic stimulates sodium reabsorption in the collecting duct. The Na^+ molecule is then exchanged for H^+ in the apical membrane. H^+ secretion is further stimulated by the increased electronegativity in the lumen of the collecting tubule at the expense of chloride. In daily practice, it can be used as an initial screening test for RTA, since it is better tolerated than the ammonium chloride test.

After emptying the bladder, 1 mg/kg furosemide is given PO. The test time duration is four hours, with sample collection at timed intervals. The lowest pH is usually reached during the third or fourth-hour collection, which is when the aforementioned volume contraction is likely to occur.

In some cases, dizziness from low blood pressure is observed. It is contraindicated in situations involving previous volume contraction clinical situations, like ADH deficiency.

The test is not accurate in patients with distal RTA, due to secretory defects and in those with voltage defects due to an impaired tubular sodium transport. In contrast, the test is normal in patients with saline loss due to aldosterone deficiency, as in type 4 renal tubular acidosis.

The urinary pH should be <5.35 to perform the test. The stimulus for the secretion of hydrogen ions produced by furosemide is lower than that of $ClNH_4$, so the titratable acid and ammonia values are lower than those obtained with furosemide [16, 26]. Therefore, the amount of ammonium excreted with this test is difficult to interpret.

In patients with idiopathic hypercalciuria, our Group has observed false-negative results with the furosemide test, since there is less excretion of titratable acid. We showed that this defect was not secondary to the possibility of resistance to the diuretic [27]. Nevertheless, the patients who did not acidify the urine using this test showed instead normal results with the pCO_2 test [26].

(b) Urinary acidification test with furosemide and fludrocortisone

In 2007, Walsh, Wrong et al. designed this test with the idea of improving the results of the furosemide acidification test, aiming to increase the secretion of H^+ ions at the cortical collecting duct [28]. The mineralocorticoid fludrocortisone mimics the action of aldosterone and activates a higher density of the epithelial sodium channels (ENaC) in the luminal membranes of the principal cells. This maneuver increases sodium reabsorption, favored by the volume contraction, as well as the secretion of ammonium by the α-intercalated cell, thereby facilitating the excretion of H^+ ions.

The activity of the basolateral Na^+K^+ATPase and H^+ATPase pumps is also increased with the administration of the mineralocorticoid in the α-intercalated cells [28, 29].

After bladder emptying, 1 mg/kg of furosemide (40 mg in adults) and fludrocortisone (1 mg/1.73 m^2) are administered PO.

Measurements, determinations, and results are the same as those described with the furosemide test. In control adults, the ammonium excretion achieved was 85 ± 23 μmol/min and the titratable acidity 42 ± 5 μmol/min, reducing the urinary pH to 4.92 ± 0.10 [28].

Shavit et al. used these tests in patients with suspected incomplete distal RTA. In 61.8% of the cases, both tests showed coincident results, but in 38.2% the furosemide-fludrocortisone test was abnormal, whereas the $ClNH_4$ test was normal [30].

Determination of Maximum Urinary pCO_2 (Stimulus to Acidify in Alkaline Urine)

In a normal situation, if there is enough concentration of urinary HCO_3^- in the collecting duct, a negative gradient is induced in the tubular lumen, and the H^+ secretion increases, producing carbonic acid (CO_3H_2). Since there is no luminal carbonic anhydrase at the distal level (unlike in the proximal tubule), the H_2CO_3 formed dissociates very slowly in H_2O and CO_2 (Fig. 7.3). If H^+ ion secretion is adequate, the CO_2 production, which is measured as pCO_2 on a gasometer, will be adequate [31–35].

In 1974, Halperin et al. confirmed that urinary pCO_2 did not rise in patients with distal RTA when subjected to CO_3HNa overload [33]. The high bicarbonate urinary excretion necessary to perform this test can be achieved with different stimuli such as sodium bicarbonate (oral or intravenous), acetazolamide, or the combination of both sodium bicarbonate with acetazolamide. It is a simple, sensitive, and well-tolerated test.

The same technique applies to the three modalities of this test. The test is done after emptying the bladder. An hour later, the patient must urinate again. Urinary pCO_2 can be measured in this sample, but better results are obtained if the sample is collected 90 minutes after the beginning of the test. When the samples are collected, the patient should be as close as possible to the laboratory where the gasometer is located. Part of the urine is withdrawn immediately through a syringe with no air bubble left on top. It is sealed with a needle that should be bend to prevent gas leakage. The urine is put into a gasometer in the same way as is done with blood

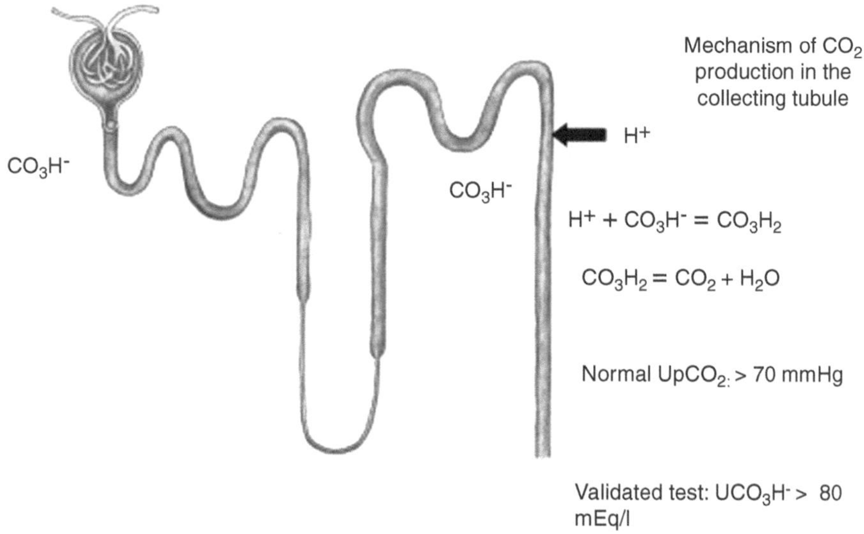

Fig. 7.3 Determination of maximum urinary pCO_2 (stimulus to acidify in alkaline urine). CO_2 production in the collecting duct

samples. The rest of the urine sample is used to determine the concentration of [Na^+] and [K^+] ions in case the gasometer does not offer a reliable result of bicarbonate excretion.

Electrolyte measurements are needed to calculate urinary bicarbonate, by Edelman's formula, as follows [14]:

$$\mathrm{UHCO_3^-} = 0.03 \times \text{urinary } \mathrm{pCO_2} \times -\log\left(\text{urinary pH} - \text{urinary pK}\right)$$

$$\text{Urinary pK}\left(\text{ionization constant}\right) =$$
$$6.33 - 0.5\left[\mathrm{UNa} + \left(\mathrm{mEq/L}\right) + \mathrm{UK} + \left(\mathrm{mEq/L}\right)\right]^{1/2}$$

For a normal result, the urinary pCO_2 must be >70 mmHg [36, 37]. The result of the test is expressed as the gradient difference between urinary/plasma pCO_2; the difference must be >30 mmHg. Furthermore, to validate the test, the bicarbonate excreted must be >80 mEq/l, which usually coincides with a urine pH >7.4–7.8 [38].

When the test is not valid (reduced bicarbonate excretion) due to a defect in the urine concentration capacity; then the [HCO_3^-]u becomes diluted. The test should be repeated, adding desmopressin simultaneously.

The test has a high specificity and sensitivity to detect defects of distal proton secretion [34]. Patients with distal RTA due to a primary defect of H^+ secretion would not be able to increase the urine pCO_2. The test is normal in cases of RTA due to permeability defect (H^+back-leak). Some cases have been reported in which urine pCO_2 is low, but NH_4^+ excretion is appropriately increased [39].

There is a myth in some hospital laboratories that urine samples cannot be inserted into the gasometers intended for blood samples. After 40 years of doing these tests in our hospital, we have never observed any problem with the different devices used. However, the introduction of samples with a pH different from the estimated range for blood can cause the apparatus to start a self-calibration process. Unless the introduction of urine samples is explicitly prohibited in the datasheet of the device, we believe that it can be used without causing any problem.

(a) Sodium bicarbonate test

Sodium bicarbonate is administered orally at the dose of 2–4 mEq/kg (1 g = 12 mEq) of sodium bicarbonate 1M is infused intravenously at a rate of 3 ml/min/1.73 m^2SA. The most frequent side effects are vomiting and abdominal pain.

(b) Acetazolamide test

Acetazolamide reduces bicarbonate reabsorption in the proximal tubule by inhibiting carbonic anhydrase, thereby promoting the arrival of bicarbonate in the distal portions of the nephron [40]. Dosing is 1 g/1.73 m^2SA, PO, or 10–15 mg/kg/dose [41, 42]. This is the least sensitive test, since the individual response is irregular and, on many occasions, low bicarbonate excretion is achieved [43]. Usually, false-negative results are more frequently obtained than, with the bicarbonate test, especially in patients with idiopathic hypercalciuria [23]. Acetazolamide is better tolerated is better than oral bicarbonate, although headaches may occur.

(c) Acetazolamide and sodium bicarbonate test

The sodium bicarbonate administered for the test is not reabsorbed in the proximal tubule due to the pharmacological effect of acetazolamide. The dose of each product is half of that indicated above for acetazolamide when given alone, so, there may be fewer side effects with both medications together [44, 45]. Sodium bicarbonate and acetazolamide are administered orally, diluted in water, at a dose of 2 mEq/kg and 500 mg/1.73 m^2 SA, respectively.

Non-significant side effects have been noticed by us in children, while in adults we have occasionally observed diarrhea, gastric discomfort, and even paresthesia. This test has been described by our Group.

Other Tests to Assess Urine Acidification by Increasing Tubular Electronegativity

Distal tubular acidification can be stimulated by increasing electronegativity at the expense of chloride (calcium chloride) [46], sulfate (sodium sulfate) [13], or phosphate overloads.

Some patients are not able to increase the urinary pCO_2 when a high bicarbonate concentration fluid is given, but they do so after the administration of phosphate. This fact has been described in secretory defects limited to the medullary proton pump [47] and in cases of voltage-dependent tubular acidosis and moderate defect of distal sodium transport. Phosphate can be administered PO or by IV infusion [48].

Study of Proximal Tubular Reabsorption of Bicarbonate (HCO_3^-)

Determination of the Renal Threshold of Bicarbonate Reabsorption

The objective of this test is to analyze the characteristics of proximal tubular HCO_3 reabsorption.

Physiologically, bicarbonate appears in the urine when blood [HCO_3^-] is above the renal tubular reabsorption threshold, while bicarbonate disappears from the urine when blood [HCO_3^-] is below the tubular threshold.

The test may be performed in patients with systemic hyperchloremic metabolic acidosis with normal distal tubular acidification capacity and, suspected isolated proximal RTA or, secondary RTA secondary to other proximal tubular defects (Toni-Debré-Fanconi syndrome).

In the case of proximal RTA, the HCO_3^- reabsorption threshold is lower than normal [49, 50]. A proximal acidification defect is suspected when the bicarbonate reabsorption threshold is lower than normal.

In newborns, the threshold is 20 mEq/l; in infants during the first year of life, the threshold ranges from 21.5 to 22.5 mEq/l [14]; in older children, between 24 and 26 mEq/l, and, in the adult population is 26 mEq/l.

Under a spontaneous metabolic acidosis, a sodium bicarbonate solution with a concentration of 0.33 mEq/ml is infused at a rate calculated to increase the $[HCO_3^-]$ around 2 mEq//h (for an approximated value of 50% of the extracellular body fluid, the rate of infusion would be 0.05 × weight (kg)/ml/min).

The bicarbonate threshold is known to have been reached when the urinary pH rises between 6.5 and 7. At this time, the infusion rate is increased 1.5 to 2 times from the previous one and maintained until the blood $[HCO_3^-]$ is increased to 25 and 30 mEq/l [14]. This test requires bladder catheterization. Urine samples are collected, under mineral oil, at half-hour intervals, to determine pH, creatinine, and bicarbonate.

In the middle of each interval, blood samples are collected to measure creatinine and a capillary blood gas analysis. Possible side effects or complications may be tetany due to alkalosis, hypokalemia, and fluid overload.

If the threshold is to be determined in a clinical situation in which the blood $[HCO_3^-]$ is not greatly decreased (> 20 mEq/l), a metabolic acidosis must be induced by ammonium chloride administration.

Bicarbonate Fractional Excretion ($FEHCO_3^-$)

The renal threshold of bicarbonate reabsorption determination is a complex and tedious test, but it allows us to have an idea of the proximal reabsorption of bicarbonate. For the diagnosis of proximal RTA, it must be confirmed that the $FEHCO_3^-$ is increased.

FE means the volume of blood (ml) that is devoid of the substance under study for every 100 ml of glomerular filtrate (GF). It determines the renal handling of the substance to be studied, by the relationship of the urine/plasma concentrations. It is equivalent to the quotient between the clearance of the studied substance and that of creatinine [51, 52]. The result is expressed in ml/100 ml of GF. No bladder catheter is required.

If metabolic acidosis is present, oral or intravenous bicarbonate is administered, depending on the base deficit at the moment [30 –plasma $[HCO_3^-]$ × body weight (kg) × 0.3]. The bladder is emptied at timed intervals. Urine creatinine and bicarbonate concentration are determined when the urine pH is >6.5–7. A blood sample is collected to quantify creatinine and a blood gas (preferably arterial) is performed to determine plasma bicarbonate levels. With these data, the EF of bicarbonate is determined using the following formula:

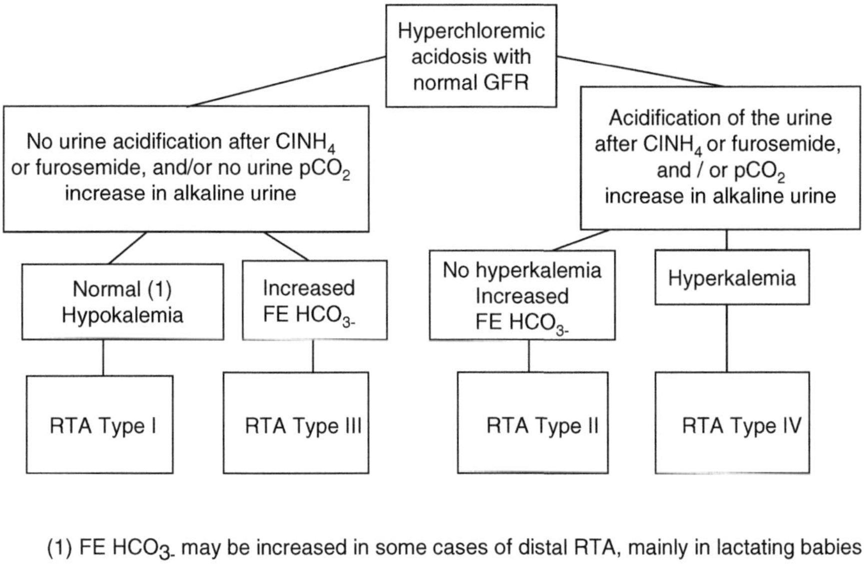

Fig. 7.4 Renal acidification tests in the four types of RTA

(urine[HCO_3^-] × plasma creatinine × 100/plasma [HCO_3^-] × urine creatinine) [16]. No bicarbonate overload is necessary if the blood [HCO_3^-] is normal.

Normal $FEHCO_3^-$ is normal with a result of <3%. When there is a proximal acidification defect, the result is >5%, and more often than not >15% (Fig. 7.4).

Epilogue The proper use of the tests narrated in this chapter allows us to distinguish the four described subtypes of RTA.

References

1. Butler AM, Wilson JL, Farber S. Dehydration and acidosis with calcification at renal tubules. J Pediatr. 1936;8:489–99.
2. Gordillo-Paniagua G. Composición orgánica. In: Electrolitos en pediatría. Fisiología y clínica. 2ª ed. México DF: Asociación de Médicos del Hospital Infantil de México; 1975. p. 39.
3. Karet FE, Gainza FJ, Györy AZ, Unwin RJ, Wrong O, Tanner MJ, et al. Mutations in the chloride-bicarbonate exchanger gene AE1 cause autosomal dominant but not autosomal recessive distal renal tubular acidosis. Proc Natl Acad Sci U S A. 1998;95:6337–42.
4. Narins RG, Emmett M. Simple and mixed acid-base disorders: a practical approach. Medicine (Baltimore). 1980;59:161–87.
5. Kraut JA, Madias NE. Serum anion gap: its uses and limitation in clinical medicine. Clin J Am Soc Nephrol. 2007;2:162–74.
6. Brennan S, Hering-Smith K, Hamm LL. Effect of pH on citrate reabsorption in the proximal convolute tubule. Am J Phys. 1988;255:F301–6.
7. Tosukhowong P, Tungsanga K, Phongudom S, Sriboonlue P. Effects of potassium-magnesium citrate supplementation on cytosolic ATP citrate lyase and mitochondrial aconitase activity in leukocytes: a window on renal citrate metabolism. Int J Urol. 2005;12:140–4.

8. Zacchia M, Preisig P. Low urinary citrate: an overview. J Nephrol. 2010;23(Suppl 16):S49–56.
9. Kraut JA, Madias NE. Differential diagnosis of nongap metabolic acidosis: value of a systematic approach. Clin J Am Soc Nephrol. 2012;7:671–9.
10. Goldstein MB, Bear R, Richardson RMA, Marsden PA, Halperin ML. The urine anion gap: a clinically useful index of ammonium excretion. Am J Med Sci. 1986;292:198–202.
11. Batlle DC, Hizon M, Cohen E, Gutterman C, Gupta R. The use of the urinary anion gap in the diagnosis of hyperchloremic metabolic acidosis. N Engl J Med. 1988;318:594–9.
12. Albright F, Consolazio WV, Coombs FS, Sulkowitch HW, Talbott JH. Metabolic studies and therapy in a case of nephrocalcinosis with rickets and dwarfism. Bull Johns Hopk Hosp. 1940;66:7–33.
13. Royer P, Mathieu H, Habib R. Acidosis tubular crónica idiopática con hipercalciuria e hipocitraturia (Síndrome de Butler-Albright). In: Problemas actuales de nefrología infantil, ed. esp. Barcelona: Ed. Toray; 1965. p. 113–25.
14. Edelmann CM Jr, Rodríguez Soriano J, Boichis H, Gruskin AB, Acosta MI. Renal bicarbonate reabsorption and hydrogen ion excretion in normal infants. J Clin Invest. 1967;46:1309–17.
15. Peonides A, Levin B, Young WF. The renal excretion of hydrogen ion in infants and children. Arch Dis Child. 1965;40:33–9.
16. García Nieto V, Santos F, Rodríguez IB. Pruebas funcionales renales. In: García Nieto V, Santos F, Rodríguez Iturbe B, editors. Nefrología Pediátrica. 2ª ed. Madrid: Aula Médica; 2006. p. 51–62.
17. Manning RT, Delp MH. Arginine hydrochloride as a system acidifier. Am J MedSci. 1961;241:575–80.
18. García Puig J, Mateos Antón F, Martínez Gómez ME, Gil Aguado A, Arnalich F, Vázquez JJ, et al. Exploración de la capacidad renal de acidificación con monoclorhidrato de L-arginina: Resultados en sujetos normales. Rev Clin Esp. 1980;156:393–8.
19. Loney LC, Norling LL, Robson AM. The use of arginine hydrochloride infusion to assess urinary acidification. J Pediatr. 1982;100:95–8.
20. Puschett JB, Goldberg M. The acute effects of furosemide on acid and electrolyte excretion in man. J Lab Clin Med. 1968;71:666–77.
21. García Puig J, Mateos Anton F, Anciones B, Grande C, Gilaquado A, Arnalich F, et al. Influencia de la furosemida sobre la disfunción acidificadora de la acidosis tubular renal. Rev Clin Esp. 1980;156:407–11.
22. Rastogi SP, Crawford C, Wheeler R, Flanigan W, Arruda JA. Effect of furosemide on urinary acidification in distal renal tubular acidosis. J Lab Clin Med. 1984;104:271–82.
23. Reynolds TM, Burgess N, Matanhelia S, Brain A, Penney MD. The frusemide test: simple screening test for renal acidification defect in urolithiasis. Br J Urol. 1993;72:153–6.
24. Kovacikova J, Winter C, Loffing-Cueni D, Loffing J, Finberg KE, Lifton RP, et al. The connecting tubule is the main site of the furosemide-induced urinary acidification by the vacuolar H+-ATPase. Kidney Int. 2006;70:1706–16.
25. Suki W, Rector FC Jr, Seldin DW. The site of action of furosemide and other sulfonamide diuretics in the dog. J Clin Invest. 1965;44:1458–69.
26. García-Nieto V, Monge M, Hernández Hernández L, Callejón A, Luis Yanes MI, García Rodríguez VE. Estudio de la capacidad de acidificación renal en niños diagnosticados de hipercalciuria idiopática. Nefrologia. 2003;23:219–24.
27. Rodríguez C, Luis Yanes MI, Delgado M, Garcia-Nieto V. ¿El defecto para acidificar la orina en la prueba realizada con furosemida, es un marcador de resistencia parcial a la acción de este fármaco? Nefrologia. 2005;25:578–9.
28. Walsh SB, Shirley DG, Wrong OM, Unwin RJ. Urinary acidification assessed by simultaneous furosemide and fludrocortisone treatment: an alternative to ammonium chloride. Kidney Int. 2007;71:1310–6.
29. Dhayat N, Gradwell M, Anderegg M, Schneider L, Luethi D, Mattmann C, et al. Furosemide/fludrocortisone test and clinical parameters to diagnose incomplete distal renal tubular acidosis in kidney stone formers. Clin J Am Soc Nephrol. 2017;12:1507–17.

30. Shavit L, Chen L, Ahmed F, Ferraro PM, Moochhala S, Walsh SB, et al. Selective screening for distal renal tubular acidosis in recurrent kidney stone formers: initial experience and comparison of the simultaneous furosemide and fludrocortisone test with the short ammonium chloride test. Nephrol Dial Transplant. 2016;31:1870–6.
31. Pitts RF, Lotspeich WD. Bicarbonate and the renal regulation of acid-base balance. Am J Phys. 1946;147:138–54.
32. Poy RK, Wrong O. The urinary pCO_2 in renal disease. Clin Sci. 1960;19:631–63.
33. Halperin ML, Goldstein MB, Haig A, Johnson MD, Stinebaugh BJ. Studies on the pathogenesis of type I (distal) renal tubular acidosis as revealed by the urinary PCO_2 tensions. J Clin Invest. 1974;53:669–77.
34. Dubose TDJR, Pucacco LR, Green JM. Hydrogen ion secretion by the collecting duct as a determinant of the urine to blood pCO_2 gradient in alkaline urine. J Clin Invest. 1982;69:145–56.
35. Kim S, Lee JW, Park J, Na KY, Joo KW, Ahn C, et al. The urine-blood PCO_2 gradient as a diagnostic index of H(+)-ATPase defect distal renal tubular acidosis. Kidney Int. 2004;66:761–7.
36. Halperin ML, Goldstein MB, Richardson RM, Stinebaugh BJ. Distal renal tubular acidosis syndromes: a pathophysiological approach. Am J Nephrol. 1985;5:1–8.
37. Peces R, Arrieta J, Batlle DC. Mecanismos y clasificación de la acidosis tubular renal. Nefrologia. 1991;11:217–23.
38. Rodríguez-Soriano J, Vallo A. Renal tubular acidosis. Pediatr Nephrol. 1990;4:268–75.
39. Vasuvattakul S, Nimmannit S, Shayakul C, Vareesangthip K, Halperin ML. Should the urine PCO2 or the rate of excretion of ammonium be the gold standard to diagnose distal renal tubular acidosis? Am J Kidney Dis. 1992;19:72–5.
40. Leaf A, Schwartz WB, Relman AS. Oral administration of a potent carbonic anhydrase inhibitor (diamox). I. Changes in electrolyte and acid-base balance. N Engl J Med. 1954;250:759–64.
41. Rubinstein H, Batlle DC, Roseman M, Sehy JT, Arruda JAL, Kurtzman NA. Urinary pCO_2 during carbonic anhydrase inhibition in the dog. Mineral Electrolyte Metab. 1981;5:49–59.
42. Alon U, Hellerstein S, Warady BA. Oral acetazolamide in the assessment of (urine-blood) PCO_2. Pediatr Nephrol. 1991;5:307–11.
43. Monge Zamorano M, García Nieto V, Espinosa Mª D, Sánchez Almeida E, Fernández González JL, León LC. ¿La prueba con estímulo de acetazolamida es útil para poder determinar la pCO_2 urinaria máxima? AnEspPediatr. 1995;42:233–4.
44. García Nieto V, Hernández-González MJ, Hernández-Hernández L, Monge M, Molini N. A new combined test to study the maximum urinary pCO_2 in the pediatric age. Pediatr Nephrol. 2002;17:C8.
45. Guerra-Hernandez NE, Ordaz-Lopez KV, Escobar-Perez L, Gomez-Tenorio C, Garcia-Nieto VM. Distal renal tubular acidosis screening by urinary acidification testing in Mexican children. Rev Investig Clin. 2015;67:191–8.
46. Brines J, Hernández R, Colomer J. Prueba corta de acidificación renal con cloruro cálcico en la infancia. AnEsp Pediatr. 1978;11:97–112.
47. Batlle D, Flores G. Underlying defects in distal renal tubular acidosis: new understandings. Am J Kidney Dis. 1996;27:896–915.
48. Vallo A, Rodríguez-Soriano J. Oral phosphate-loading test for the assessment of distal urinary acidification in children. Mineral Electrolyte Metab. 1984;10:387–90.
49. Rodríguez Soriano J, Boichis H, Stark H, Edelmann CM Jr. Proximal renal tubular acidosis. A defect in bicarbonate reabsorption with normal urinary acidification. Pediatr Res. 1967;1:81–98.
50. Igarashi T, Sekine T, Inatomi J, Seki G. Unraveling the molecular pathogenesis of isolated proximal renal tubular acidosis. J Am Soc Nephrol. 2002;13:2171–7.
51. Santos F, García Nieto V. Función renal basal. En: Nefrología Pediátrica, 2ª ed. García Nieto V, Santos F, Rodríguez Iturbe B, eds. Madrid: Aula Médica 2006, pp. 39–49.
52. Nguyen MT, Maynard SE, Kimmel PL. Misapplications of commonly used kidney equations: renal physiology in practice. Clin J Am Soc Nephrol. 2009;4:528–34.

Chapter 8
Proximal Renal Tubular Acidosis (Type II)

Mara Medeiros, Omar Guadarrama, and Ricardo Muñoz

Introduction

In theory, proximal renal tubular acidosis (RTA) should have been depicted as Type I RTA since the alteration is located in the proximal tubule. However, distal renal tubular acidosis or Type I RTA was the first to be described. Therefore, chronologically, the corresponding place of proximal RTA is Type II or PRTA [1, 2].

According to the etiology, PRTA may be primary or secondary. In turn, PRTA can be sub-classified as hereditary, congenital, or acquired.

M. Medeiros (✉)
Research and Diagnosis of Nephrology and, Bone Mineral Metabolism, Hospital Infantil de México Federico Gómez, Mexico City, Mexico

Faculty of Medicine, National Autonomous University of Mexico, Mexico City, Mexico

National System of Investigators, Level III, Mexico City, Mexico

O. Guadarrama
Research and Diagnosis of Nephrology and, Bone Mineral Metabolism, Hospital Infantil de México Federico Gómez, Mexico City, Mexico

R. Muñoz
Retired from: Department of Pediatric Nephrology, Hemodialysis Unit, The Children's Hospital at Albany Medical Center, Albany, NY, USA

Retired from: Pediatric Nephrology Department, Hospital Infantil de México Federico Gómez, Mexico City, Mexico

Retired from: Research Division, Hospital Infantil de Mexico Federico Gomez, Mexico City, Mexico

Retired from: National System of Investigators, Level I, Mexico City, Mexico

Retired from: North American Pediatric Renal Transplantation Collaborative Study (NAPRTCS) Study, Woburn, MA, USA

R. Muñoz (ed.), *Renal Tubular Acidosis in Children*,
https://doi.org/10.1007/978-3-030-91940-5_8

Secondary PRTA becomes part of a systemic primary disease, which, in addition to the RTA-related abnormalities, other clinical and laboratory manifestations may appear, secondary to multiple functional alterations present in the proximal tubule.

The clinical presentation of PRTA is a syndrome characterized by a hyperchloremic systemic metabolic acidosis, with a normal anion gap, hypokalemia, rickets, anorexia, vomiting, and failure to thrive. In most cases, the concentration of bicarbonate in the blood $[HCO_3^-]_s$ is usually around 15 mmol/l. In most cases of PRTA secondary to systemic diseases, the more conspicuous symptoms are dependent upon the primary disease. Symptoms of the primary disease overlap and tend to predominate over the symptoms of the RTA. This knowledge is relevant, since misdiagnosing the systemic primary disease or, the secondary RTA, may lead to establishing an erroneous treatment, thus hindering adequate care of the patient [3, 4].

Etiology and Pathophysiology

In a normal adult under physiological conditions, the filtered bicarbonate, approximately 4000 mmol daily, is almost completely reabsorbed in the proximal tubule ($\cong$ 90%). The rest is reabsorbed in the distal nephron, so the final urine is HCO_3^- free.

The proximal tubule performs two basic tubular functions which keep the balance of acid-base metabolism. The first consists of the synthesis and tubular secretion of ammonia (NH_3), which once in the tubular lumen captures an H^+ ion to become ammonium (NH_4^+). The buffer solution called ammonia contains both compounds, ammonia and ammonium (NH_3/NH_4^+), with a pK $\cong$ 9.2. In the tubular lumen of the nephron, the greatest amount of ammonia is NH_4^+. The excretion of hydrogen ions by the buffer system ammonia/ammonium is the most effective physiological method of H^+ excretion from the extracellular fluid (ECF). The counterpart, titratable acid, mainly phosphoric acid and, sulfuric acid, with their corresponding bases (HPO_4=/$H_2PO_4^-$ and HSO_4=/H_2SO_4), takes care of excreting about the other half of the total amount of H^+ eliminated by the kidneys.

On the other hand, during an episode of systemic metabolic acidosis (whatever the etiology), most of the H^+ ions (protons) are excreted as ammonia. The excretion of H^+ ions free of a buffer solution, either as ammonia or titratable acid, represents only a small amount of the total excretion of hydrogen ions from the ECF, with little importance to the whole acid-base metabolism. Nonetheless, urinary-free H^+ ions determine the pH of the urine [5].

The second important function of the proximal tubule is the recovery of the filtered bicarbonate. (See Chap. 2).

The bicarbonate of the glomerular filtrate present in the lumen as a molecule of $Na^+HCO_3^-$ cannot undergo reabsorption as such in the proximal tubule, so the molecule must dissociate in sodium and bicarbonate. The Na^+ molecule gets reabsorbed in the apical membrane of the brush border cells, in exchange for H^+, in the presence of the exchanger Na^+/H^+ (NHE 3). Then, the sodium reabsorption continues in the basolateral membrane into the peritubular space and *vasa recta*, by the action of the antiporter Na^+K^+ATPase at this site [6–8].

The bicarbonate remaining in the tubular lumen (previously secreted at the apical membrane by NHE3) binds to an H^+ molecule to form carbonic acid (H_2CO_3). Carbonic acid then breaks down into H_2O and CO_2 in the presence of the extracellular enzyme carbonic anhydrase-IV. Both molecules are reabsorbed into the cytosol by the action of aquaporins, which have the transmembrane capacity to transport both, water and gas; in this case CO_2 molecules. Again, once in the cytosol of the proximal tubular cell, the Na^+ and HCO_3^- molecules, in the presence of intracellular carbonic anhydrase II (AC II), reassemble to form $Na^+HCO_3^-$, which will be reabsorbed through the basolateral membrane via the NBC1 cotransporter [9–11].

Proximal RTA is characterized by a defect in the proximal tubular function, due to a low threshold for bicarbonate reabsorption. Several pathological situations may cause this alteration, which is analyzed below. It should be noted that the reduction in the proximal reabsorption of HCO_3^- increases its distal tubular load, exceeding the tubular HCO_3^- reabsorption capacity in this latter segment, with an increase in urinary bicarbonate excretion, thus ensuing a secondary increase in the urinary pH.

However, the distal acidification capacity is intact in patients with PRTA. Therefore, when the plasma concentration of bicarbonate [HCO_3^-] decreases and equals the reduced threshold of the proximal reabsorption, the distal portion of the tubule increases the reabsorption of bicarbonate and the excretion of H^+, until the urinary acidification capacity at the distal level has been recovered, with reduction of the urinary pH to ≤ 5.5 [12]. This may happen when the patient with PRTA develops extra-renal losses of bicarbonate, such as in patients having diarrhea. Under these clinical circumstances and given the physiological adaptations mentioned, contrary to what happens in patients with distal RTA, the patients with proximal RTA may be able to acidify the urine.

Clinical Aspects

The clinical presentation and pathophysiology of PRTA depend on the etiology of the defect of the mechanism of renal tubular reabsorption of HCO_3^-. Hence, PRTA may be sporadic, hereditary (autosomal recessive or dominant), or acquired.

Specific inherited chromosome mutations do not show clinically with Fanconi's syndrome.

Isolated primary RTA occurs sporadically or as hereditary. The clinical presentation is the usual signs and symptoms of RTA, without any other clinical manifestations [13]. However, this presentation is infrequent among the RTAs. All types of RTA are rare in the holistic concept of kidney disease in Pediatrics. Furthermore, the primary or inherited forms of ATR Type IV are even rarer than the acquired forms.

The most frequent form of hereditary proximal RTA is the recessive type, in which there are mutations of the cotransporter $Na^+HCO_3^-$ or NBCe1 (gene SLC4A4,

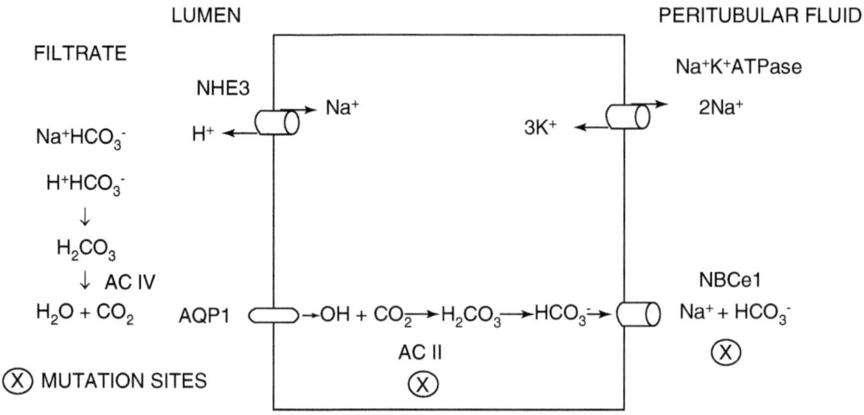

Fig. 8.1 Chromosomal alterations in hereditary pRTA. The X mark indicates the molecules with chromosomal alterations, which are found in the intracellular carbonic anhydrase II (AC II) enzyme of the brush border cells of the proximal tubule. This enzyme accelerates the equilibrium reaction, in the hydration phase of the equilibrium reaction to form carbonic acid (H_2CO_3) and Na^+ + HCO_3^-. The other molecule that is pointed out is the Na^+/HCO_3^- exchanger, called NBCe1, which undergoes mutations in the SL4A4/4q21 chromosome. This latter molecule reabsorbs sodium bicarbonate through the basolateral membrane of the proximal tubule

chromosome 4p21), which seems to have a stoichiometry of 3 HCO_3^-:1 Na^+. The clinical manifestations appear at an early age; in addition to metabolic acidosis with hyperchloremia and hypokalemia, failure to thrive, severe ocular disorders (glaucoma, band keratopathy, cataracts), cerebral calcifications (mainly in the basal ganglia), mental retardation, hypothyroidism, and dental, as well as pancreatic alterations, may also be present. This type of proximal RTA was initially described in Japan [11, 14, 15]. (See Chap. 2, Fig. 8.1).

Another rare variety of hereditary PRTA is the mutation of the intracellular carbonic anhydrase II enzyme (CA II gene, chromosome 8q22) (See Chap. 4). Since AC II is expressed in the proximal and distal tubules, deficiency of this enzyme shows clinically as mixed RTA or Type III. Genetic transmission is autosomal recessive, with osteopetrosis secondary to osteoclastic disorders and mental retardation. Nowadays, most authors considered mixed or Type III RTA, to be a sub-classification of distal RTA, instead of an isolated specific pathology.

There may be systemic manifestations due to the wide distribution of AC II in the body [16, 17]. There are 15 known forms of AC, being AC II the most conspicuously distributed in the human body. Also, it has the highest catalytic activity [18].

The autosomal dominant form of PRTA has only been described in two families, one in Costa Rica, whose affected individuals had failure to thrive and rickets [19, 20]. Most cases of PRTA are secondary to rare systemic diseases of diverse etiology, presenting clinically as Fanconi's syndrome, with glycosuria, aminoaciduria, citraturia, phosphaturia, calcinuria, low-grade proteinuria and, RTA, with urinary bicarbonate loss, among other manifestations.

According to their frequency, most of these pathologies are rare or very rare in children. Secondary RTA is not always present. These diseases are sporadic or inherited, like those of the intermediate metabolism, tubulointerstitial nephritis of various etiologies, induced by the use of nephrotoxic drugs (analgesics, antibiotics), lupus nephropathy, Sjögren's disease, Wilson's disease, kidney diseases: medullary cystic, cystinosis, galactosemia, tyrosinemia, hereditary fructose intolerance, Lowe's syndrome, von Gierke's disease, Fanconi-Bickel syndrome, Dent's disease, etc. In recent times, PRTA has been described during HIV antiviral treatment; hepatitis, and in patients with kidney transplantation (±20%). The symptoms depend on the etiology. However, most patients manifest clinically as Fanconi's syndrome [21].

Nephropathic cystinosis is an inherited metabolic disorder. In Mexico, it is one of the diseases in children that most frequently presents with proximal RTA and clinically manifestations of Fanconi's syndrome. Even so, it is classified as rare in our country, since its incidence is 1:100,000–1: 200,000 births, according to the December 2017 report from FEMEXER (Mexican Federation of Rare Diseases). The genetic mutation is located at the CTNS gene (chromosome 17p13), which encodes the cystinosine protein, apparently a lysosomal membrane protein, whose function is that of a cystine-specific membrane lysosomal transporter, with systemic distribution [22]. The organs most affected are the eyes (with cystine deposits in the anterior chamber of the eyeballs) and the kidneys (nephropathic cystinosis, with cystine deposits in the lysosomes) [23, 24]. The accumulation of lysosomal cystine in the brush border cells of the renal proximal tubule produces tubular atrophy with the light microscopy appearance described as "gooseneck", lesions that lead to the development of Fanconi's syndrome [25]. Clinical signs are those of hypothyroidism, failure to thrive, hypophosphatemic rickets, and impaired renal function. There is progression to chronic renal failure without specific treatment [26].

Some immunological diseases, like systemic lupus erythematosus (SLE), may also course with PRTA. SLE is a disease of unknown origin, characterized by the production of autoantibodies, such as antinuclear, antiphospholipid, antimitochondrial antibodies, etc.

SLE may involve the kidneys (lupus nephropathy), with progressive reduction of the glomerular filtration rate (GFR), proteinuria, and proximal RTA. The incidence of SLE is more frequently seen in children than adults, and also the clinical presentation is more aggressive. According to the international literature, the incidence of SLE is 1–20:900,000 children. In these cases, the development of lupus nephropathy is <100,000 (children/year), with morbidity of 3.3–24:100,000 children/year [26]. The incidence is greater in females (8–13:1) [27].

In an extensive population of North American children, an average annual incidence of systemic lupus erythematosus is 2.22 (95% confidence index [CI]: 2.05–2.40) and the incidence of lupus nephropathy was 0.72 (95% CI 0.63–0.83) cases/100,000 children between 3 and 18 years of age, while the prevalence of SLE was 9.73 (95% CI: 9.38–10.08)/100,000 children, and the prevalence of lupus nephropathy was 3.64 (95% CI 3.43–3.86)/100,000 children [28].

The clinical presentation of SLE is similar to the adults but differs in terms of the repercussions on growth and development, failure in school performance, psychological disturbances due to the presence of a chronic disease, which may be aggravated by the presence of lupus encephalopathy, and when kidney damage is progressive, mainly when substitute therapies for kidney function are needed [29].

Contrary to the adult population, most children with SLE (60–80%) show symptoms of Lupus Nephropathy at the onset of the disease [30]. Histopathological findings in the kidney tissue obtained by biopsy and studied by light microscopy, immunofluorescence, and electron microscopy show variable types of lesions. The results are classified according to the World Health Organization (WHO).

Study groups of the renal histopathological lesions have described six degrees of the alterations. Grade IV is characterized by changes compatible with diffuse exudative endocapillary and extracapillary glomerulonephritis, showing various types of immune complex deposits located in the glomerular tuft and the renal tubules. Also, extracapillary deposits with crescents formation, accompanied by acute proliferative inflammatory lesions, may be reversible with the appropriate treatment, contrary to the presence of chronic, usually non-reversible fibrotic lesions [31].

These latter severe histopathological lesions are associated with poorer evolution, with a rapid progression to end-stage renal failure. Since more than half the children with lupus nephropathy present this type of injury in the initial renal biopsy, the prognosis is more severe than in the adult patients [32].

The clinical findings of lupus nephropathy are related to the development of glomerulonephritis with acute nephritic syndrome or nephritic-nephrotic syndrome, characterized by hypertension, hypocomplementemia, hematuria, proteinuria, edema, and azotemia. PRTA may appear in patients with SLE, with the usual signs and symptoms.

Lab immunological studies show hypocomplementemia, specific autoantibodies, such as anti-DNA; anti-nuclear; anti-phospholipid antibodies, etc. [33].

The urinary sediment show free red and white blood cells, with red and white blood cell casts, usually accompanied by granular, waxy, and hyaline cells.

Nephrotoxicity from diverse drugs and medications is another acquired form of PRTA, usually reversible when the toxic drug is discontinued, as soon as possible after detection of the toxicity.

In some clinical situations, toxic substances may produce tubular lesions, such as membrane thin-chain disease, amyloidosis, myeloma, autoimmune diseases, as well as the intake of toxic metals such as cadmium, lead, mercury, gold, and bismuth.

The drugs more frequently associated with nephrotoxicity are antibiotics, analgesics, non-steroidal anti-inflammatory drugs, x-ray contrast media, hypertonic solutions, anesthetics, chemotherapy, calcineurin inhibitors, etc.

Some medications associated with the development of PRTA include carbonic anhydrase-inhibitors (acetazolamide), ifosfamide, topiramate, aminoglycosides, valproic acid, tenofovir, ritonavir, etc. [34–36].

Some predisposing risk factors associated with the development of nephrotoxicity should be identified and included in the clinical chart, like the health status of the individual at the time, and pre-existing illnesses, before the administration of the drug in question (kidney failure, liver disease, diabetes, hydration status, hypovolemia), age of the patient (newborn, prematurity, childhood, senescence), administration of multiple nephrotoxic drugs, specific toxicity of each drug, synergism, and genetic polymorphisms, among others. Besides, it is important to mention that the nephrotoxicity of the drugs increases with a concomitant reduction of the renal blood flow, which under normal situations is 20–25% of the effective cardiac output [37].

The clinical manifestations vary, since the drug's nephrotoxicity renders multiple histopathological alterations, such as tubular necrosis, cortical necrosis, tubulointerstitial nephritis, leukocyte accumulation with the presence of eosinophils, and so on. Oliguria, albuminuria, RBCs, hyaline, and granular casts may appear in the urine sediment. Azotemia, acute and chronic renal injury, as well as renal tubular acidosis, generally proximal or distal, may appear [37, 38]. Therefore, during the evaluation of plausible nephrotoxicity, the questions asked must be directed to detect the administration of potentially nephrotoxic drugs. The diagnosis is confirmed by laboratory studies, such as CBC, blood chemistry, electrolytes, glomerular filtration rate, urinalysis, electrolytes in the urine, albuminuria, etc. Radiological studies may include abdominal x-rays, renal ultrasound, and urinary tract. Other laboratory studies may be indicated in agreement with the suspected diagnosis, including sometimes a percutaneous kidney biopsy.

Several biomarkers have recently been studied in blood and urine, such as the "lipocalin-associated neutrophil gelatinase" (NGAL), the transmembrane protein "kidney damage molecule-1" (KIM-1), interleukins (IL-18), the "protein fatty acid binding" (L-FABP), and cardiac fatty acid binding protein (HFABP), cyclophilins, α1-microglobulin, β2-microglobulin, and clusterines, among others. These biomarkers, mainly performed in the urine, are intended to support the detection of renal proximal tubular damage. To date, no marker detects the presence of proximal RTA, becoming very important to make the proper diagnosis of this condition with the usual methods at hand, up to this time, and avoiding over-diagnosis of this entity [39].

References

1. Lightwood R. Calcium infarction of the kidneys in infants. Arch Dis Child. 1935;10:205–6.
2. Soriano JR. Renal tubular acidosis: the clinical entity. J Am Soc Nephrol. 2002;13(8):2160–70.
3. Hamm LL, Nakhoul N, Hering-Smith KS. Acid-base homeostasis. Clin J Am Soc Nephrol. 2015;10(12):2232–42.
4. Reddy P, Mooradian AD. Clinical utility of anion gap in deciphering acid-base disorders. Int J Clin Pract. 2009;63(10):1516–25.
5. Weiner ID, Hamm LL. Molecular mechanisms of renal ammonia transport. Annu Rev Physiol. 2007;69:317–40.
6. Burckhardt G, DiSole F, Helmle-Kolb C. The Na^+/H^+ exchanger gene family. J Nephrol. 2002;15(Suppl 5):S3–S21.
7. Wang T, Hropor M, Aronson PS, Giebisch G. Role of NHE isoforms in mediating bicarbonate reabsorption along the nephron. Am J Phys. 2001;281:F1120–8.
8. Jorgensen PL. Structure, function and, regulation of Na+, K+-ATPase in the kidney. Kidney Int. 1986;29:10–20.

9. Nielsen S, Agre P. The aquaporin family of water channels. Kidney Int. 1995;48(4):1057–106.
10. Silverman DN, Lindskoo S. The catalytic mechanism of carbonic anhydrase: implications of a rate-limiting protolysis of water. Acc Chem Res. 1988;21(1):30–6.
11. Soleimani M. $Na^{+}HCO_3$ cotransporter (NBC): expression and regulation in the kidney. J Nephrol. 2002;(Suppl 5):S32–40.
12. Alpern RJ. Renal acidification mechanisms. In: Brenner BM, editor. Brenner & Rector's the kidney. 6th ed. Philadelphia: W. B. Saunders Company; 2000. p. 455–519.
13. Roth KS, Chan JMC. Renal tubular acidosis: a new look at an old problem. Clin Pediatr. 2001;40:533–43.
14. Igarashi T, Inatomi J, Sekine T, Seki G, Shimadzu M, Tozawa F, Takeshima Y, Takumi T, Takahashi T, Yoshikawa N, Nakamura H, Endou H. Novel nonsense mutation in the Na+/HCO3- cotransporter gene (SLC4A4) in a patient with permanent isolated proximal renal tubular acidosis and bilateral glaucoma. J Am Soc Nephrol. 2001;12:713–8.
15. Romero MF, Boron WF. Electrogenic Na+/HCO3- cotransporters: cloning and physiology. Annu Rev Physiol. 1999;61:699–723.
16. Whyte MP, Murphy WA, Fallon MD, Sly WS, Teitelbaum SL, McAlister WH, et al. Osteopetrosis, renal tubular acidosis and, basal ganglia calcification in three sisters. Am J Med. 1980;69:64–74.
17. Strisciuglio P, Sartorio R, Pecoraro C, Lotito F, Sly WS. Variable clinical presentation of carbonic anhydrase deficiency: evidence for heterogeneity? Eur J Pediatr. 1990;149:337–40.
18. Baird TT, Waheed A, Okuyama T, et al. Catalysis and inhibition of human carbonic anhydrase IV. Biochemistry. 1997;36:2669–78.
19. Brenes LG, Brenes JN, Hernandez MM. Familial proximal renal tubular acidosis. A distinct clinical entity. Am J Med. 1977;63:244–52.
20. Lemann J Jr, Adams ND, Wilz DR, Brenes LG. Acid and mineral balances and bone in familial proximal renal tubular acidosis. Kidney Int. 2000;58:1267–77. https://doi.org/10.1046/j.1523-1755.2000.00282.x.
21. Haque SK, Ariceta G, Batlle D. Proximal renal tubular acidosis: a not so rare disorder of multiple etiologies. Nephrol Dial Transplant. 2012;27(12):4273–87. https://doi.org/10.1093/ndt/gfs493, PMCID: PMC3616759 PMID: 23235953.
22. Gahl WA, Thoene JG, Schneider JA. Cystinosis: a disorder of lysosomal membrane transport. In: Scriver CR, Beaudet AL, Sly WS, Valle D, editors. The metabolic and molecular bases of inherited disease, vol. 3. 8th ed. New York: McGraw Hill; 2001. p. 5085–108.
23. Town M, Jean G, Cherqui S, et al. A novel gene encoding an integral membrane protein is mutated in nephropathic cystinosis. Nat Genet. 1998;18:319–24.
24. Kalatzis V, Cherqui S, Antignac C, Gasnier B. Cystinosin, the protein defective in cystinosis, is an H -driven lysosomal cystine transporter. EMBO J. 2001;20:5940–9.
25. Pintos M. Cistinosisnefropática. Nefrología. 2011;2(1):1–119. Suplemento Extraordinario.pre 2011. https://doi.org/10.3265/Mar.10910.
26. Mahoney CP, Striker GE. Early development of the renal lesions in infantile cystinosis. Pediatr Nephrol. 2000;15:50–6.
27. Mina R, Brunner HI. Update on differences between childhood-onset and adult-onset systemic lupus erythematosus 2013. Arthritis Res Therapy. 2013;15:218.
28. Hiraki LT, Feldman J, Alarcón GS, Fisher MA, Winkelmayer WC, Costenbader KH. Prevalence, incidence and, demographics of systemic lupus erythematosus and lupus nephritis among Medicaid-enrolled U.S. children, 2000–2004. Arthritis Rheum. 2012;64(8):2669–76. https://doi.org/10.1002/art.34472.
29. Klein-Gitelman M, Reiff A, Silverman ED. Systemic lupus erythematosus in childhood. Rheum Dis Clin N Am. 2002;(28):561–77.
30. Bakkaloglu A. Lupus nephropathy in children. Nephrol Dial Transplant. 2001;16(Suppl 6):126–8.

31. Zappitelli M, Duffy C, Bernard C, Scuccimarri R, Duffy KW, Kagan R, Gupta IR. Clinicopathological study of the WHO classification in childhood lupus nephritis. Pediatr Nephrol. 2004;19:503–10.
32. Weening JJ, D'Agati VD, Schwartz MM, Seshan SV, Alpers CE, Appel GB, et al. The classification of glomerulonephritis in systemic lupus erythematosus revisited. Kidney Int. 2004;(6565):521–30.
33. Gallego N y Col. Nefropatía lúpica en la infancia: estudio multicéntrico. Nefrología. 1999:(19):0–390.
34. Dharmarajan L, Ammar H. Expanding the differential: toluene-induced toxicity. BMJ Case Rep. 2017;2017:bcr-2017.
35. Weiner SM. Renal involvement in connective tissue diseases. Dtsch Med Wochenschr. 2018;143(2):89–100.
36. Gupta S, Gao JJ, Emmett M, Fenves AZ. Topiramate and metabolic acidosis: an evolving story. Hosp Pract (1995). 2017;45(5):192–5.
37. Sari A. Nephrotoxic effects of drugs, poisoning in the modern world – new tricks for an old dog? OzgurKarcioglu and Banu Arslan, IntechOpen; 2019. https://doi.org/10.5772/intechopen.83644. Available from: https://www.intechopen.com/books/poisoning-in-the-modern-world-new tricks-for-an-old-dog-/nephrotoxic-effects-of-drugs.
38. Striker LJ, Olson JL, Striker GE. Tubular and interstitial lesions. In: Striker LJ, Olson JL, Striker GE, editors. The renal biopsy. Philadelphia: WB Saunders Company; 1990. p. 254–70.
39. Stephen W, Waring WS, Moonie A. Earlier recognition of nephrotoxicity using novel biomarkers of acute kidney injury. J Clin Toxicol. 2011;49:720–8.

Chapter 9
Distal Renal Tubular Acidosis (Type I DRTA)

Ricardo Muñoz

Introduction

DRTA was initially described as a clinical entity by Lightwood [1] and later on by Rodríguez-Soriano [2] designated it as the first type of renal tubular acidosis, called at that time classic, distal, or type I RTA.

On the other hand, proximal RTA was described chronologically in the second place and, thus named type II RTA.

DRTA is the most frequent type of renal tubular acidosis in the pediatric age group. However, similarly to other types of RTA, it is a rare entity worldwide. The epidemiology of type I RTA is discussed in more detail in Chap. 4 of this book.

According to the etiology, DRTA is classified as primary or secondary. The latter is a companion of several systemic diseases or secondary to the administration of certain potentially nephrotoxic drugs, such as amphotericin B, toluene, lithium, trimethoprim, ifosfamide, foscarnet, analgesics, and so on.

Certain clinical entities, such as medullary sponge kidney disease and, some diseases of autoimmune etiology, may be the cause of secondary DRTA:

R. Muñoz (✉)
Retired from: Department of Pediatric Nephrology, Hemodialysis Unit, The Children's Hospital at Albany Medical Center, Albany, NY, USA

Retired from: Pediatric Nephrology Department, Hospital Infantil de México Federico Gómez, Mexico City, Mexico

Retired from: Research Division, Hospital Infantil de Mexico Federico Gomez, Mexico City, Mexico

Retired from: National System of Investigators, Level I, Mexico City, Mexico

Retired from: North American Pediatric Renal Transplantation Collaborative Study (NAPRTCS) Study, Woburn, MA, USA

R. Muñoz (ed.), *Renal Tubular Acidosis in Children*,
https://doi.org/10.1007/978-3-030-91940-5_9

hypergammaglobulinemia, Sjögren's syndrome, disseminated lupus erythematosus, rheumatoid arthritis, and polyarteritis nodosa, among others [3, 4]. Some of these diseases are discussed in the corresponding chapters.

Pathophysiology of Hereditary DRTA

Historically, the pathophysiology of DRTA has gone through various scientific theories and hypotheses, mainly due to the technological advances available in each era, a process that will continue with the development of newer knowledge.

Traditionally, it is nowadays considered that the functional alteration in the proximal RTA (type II) is a defect in the bicarbonate reabsorption, whereas in DRTA (type I) there is a reduced ability of urinary acidification located in the distal tubule.

Nevertheless, these functional alterations overlap, since the proximal tubule retains a certain acidification capacity, whereas the collecting tubule may produce and reabsorb some amount of bicarbonate. Therefore, the classification is mainly based on the primary dominant function of each segment of the nephron.

The highest excretion of H^+ takes place in the connecting and collecting tubules, by buffer systems acting as titratable acid and ammonia and, as a consequence, the formation and reabsorption of new bicarbonate [5].

DRTA is currently considered to be the result of renal alterations in the capacity to acidify the urine, in turn, being secondary to a dysfunction of the α-intercalated cells of the collecting tubules.

All these functional alterations obey specific chromosomal mutations of the transporter proteins that translocate H^+ ions transmembrane at the α-intercalated cells. H^+ ions are mainly transported as ammonium (NH_4^+) and bicarbonate (HCO_3^-) molecules.

The chromosomal mutations lead to the development of DRTA, usually in the absence, or just with a slight reduction of the glomerular filtration rate (GFR).

Nonetheless, some cases may show a small reduction in the filtration rate that, when it happens, is discordant with the degree of metabolic acidosis.

By reducing the distal tubular excretion of protons in the form of buffering compounds, mainly phosphates and sulfates (titratable acid) and ammonia/ammonium (NH_3/NH_4^+), the formation and reabsorption of bicarbonate is reduced. Consequently, the serum bicarbonate concentration $[HCO_3^-]s$ is reduced and hyperchloremic systemic metabolic acidosis with a normal anion gap develops [6].

The fine regulation of acid-base metabolism at the end of the nephron takes place in the α-intercalated cells of the connecting and collecting tubules. Transporter proteins of H^+ and HCO_3^- take care of this function, such as H^+ATPase (hydrogen adenosine triphosphatase (ATP), also called vacuolar H^+ATPase (VH^+ ATPase) or "hydrogen pump". This transporter protein performs the highest excretion of cytosolic H^+ through the apical membrane of the α-intercalated cells toward the distal tubular lumen, where H^+ ions are entrapped, to be excreted subsequently in the final urine as titratable acid and ammonia. This function is independent of Na^+ distal tubular reabsorption.

Albeit indirectly, Na^+ reabsorption at this level participates in the final excretion of H^+, since the antiporter Na^+/K^+ pump (Na^+/K^+ATPase), expressed in the basolateral membrane affects the role of H^+ ATPase through changes in the transmembrane electrical potential facilitating the distal excretion of H^+ [7].

The hydrogen/potassium pump (H^+K^+ ATPase) transporter protein, located in the apical membrane of the α-intercalated cells, also intervenes in the distal excretion of H^+, although to a lesser extent than H^+ ATPase, since the H^+K^+ATPase pump responds mainly to changes in the [K^+] of the extracellular fluid space (ECF). This physiological mechanism, in turn, depends on the action of aldosterone. To date, no chromosomal abnormalities have been detected in H^+K^+ATPase, which could lead to the development of distal RTA.

HCO_3^- is reabsorbed in the basolateral membrane from the cytosol into the peritubular fluid and *vasa recta*, by the anion exchanger AE1, which exchanges HCO_3^- for Cl^-. The AE1 anion exchanger is expressed in various organs; in the kidney, it is called kAE1 [8, 9].

The function of the vacuolar H^+ATPase at the apical membrane of the α-intercalated cell is linked to the physiology of the kAE1 exchanger, for the reabsorption of bicarbonate. This function is favored by the intracellular carbonic anhydrase catalytic metalloenzyme (AC II), which participates in the process of cellular respiration and accelerates the rate of the equilibrium reaction in the hydration of CO_2 to form carbonic acid (H_2CO_3) and, at the end of the reaction, to HCO_3^- and H^+. AC II is the source of intracellular production of HCO_3^-, which is reabsorbed in the basolateral membrane by the HCO_3^-/Cl^- antitransporter (kAE1) to the systemic circulation toward the extracellular fluid space (ECF), as new bicarbonate. During the intracellular equilibrium reaction, protons are produced and excreted in the apical membrane toward the tubular lumen by the vacuolar H^+ATPase [10]. The H^+ molecules are excreted in the final urine accompanied by a buffer, mainly titratable acid, which is made up of various compounds, mainly phosphates (HPO_4^{-2}/HPO_4^-), with pK 6.80, plus sulfates (HPO_4^{-2}/HPO_4^-), as well as ammonia, consisting of the buffer pair ammonia and ammonium (NH_3/NH_4^+), with pK $\cong$ 9.3.

H^+ and K^+ can be exchanged for NH_4^+ molecules at the membrane sites of the transporter proteins H^+ATPase, H^+K^+ ATPase and, Na^+/K^+ATPase, for excretion of NH_4^+ in the final urine. Other important transporter proteins for the excretion of ammonia in the α-intercalated cells in the collecting tubules are the Rhesus (Rh) glycoproteins: Rhcg and Rhbg, as well as the "cationic channels activated by hyperpolarization and cyclic nucleotides" (HCN), also called "pacemaker channels" [11–13]. The physiological mechanisms of H^+ secretion and excretion participating in the renal regulation of acid-base metabolism are reviewed in detail in Chap. 2.

The genetic mutations that give rise to the primary or hereditary DRTA are located in the α-intercalated cells of the connecting and collecting tubules and explain the pathophysiology of this entity [14]. To date, three chromosomal mutations have been described, including the H^+ secreting protein (vacuolar H^+ATPase), the HCO_3^-/CL^- anion exchanger (AE1), and intracellular AC II. See Fig. 9.1.

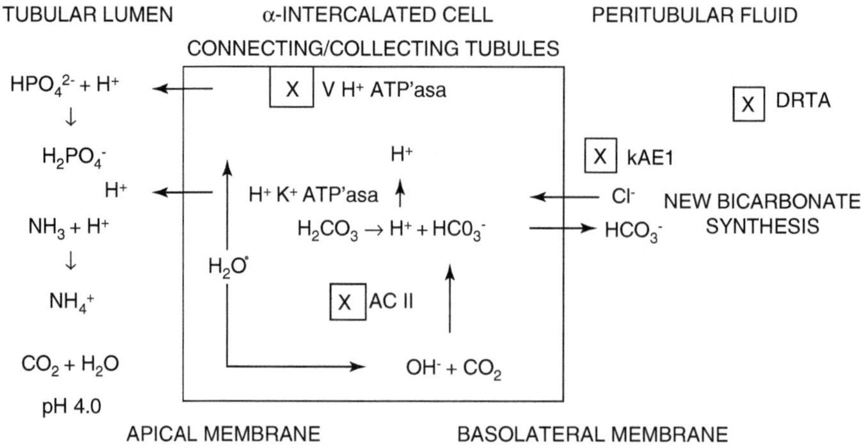

Fig. 9.1 Mark X indicates the sites of the chromosomal alterations of primary (hereditary) DRTA. They are located in the α-intercalated cells in the collecting tubules. The anionic antiporter kAE1 exchanges HCO_3^-/Cl^- at the basolateral membrane. The H-V ATPase transporter secrets hydrogen ions from the cytosol to the distal tubular lumen. Intracellular AC II is expressed in both, proximal and distal tubules, where the equilibrium reaction reverts the site of hydration of CO_2, for its conversion to H_2CO_3 and, in turn, to $H^+ + HCO_3^-$. The bicarbonate molecule is reabsorbed through the basolateral membrane by the kAE1 antiporter and, from there, shifted to the ECF

The heterogeneity of the hereditary pattern, as well as the variations of the clinical presentation, is not due to a complete functional absence. Instead, they are due to specific functional deficiencies secondary to mutations in the genes involved. Furthermore, the function of the molecules can be altered by different mechanisms, such as failure of the intracellular trafficking of the affected protein, sequestration of the protein in the organelles, or due to the protein's inability to recognize the target organ.

The inherited pattern of the involved genetic mutations can be autosomal dominant or recessive. This becomes relevant to genetic counseling, as well as to have a better idea about the penetration of the gen and, the severity of the clinical presentation of RTA [15].

The genetic mutations, hereditary patterns, and clinical presentation are described below.

Chromosomal and Physiological Alterations of the AE1 Antiporter

The AE1 exchanger, which exchanges HCO_3^-/Cl^-, belongs to the SCL4A1 gene family; is encoded on chromosome 17q 1-22 and is expressed in different organs and tissues, such as the basolateral membrane of α-intercalated cells of the connecting and collecting tubules in the cortical and medullary regions, as well as in the plasma membrane of erythrocytes [16, 17].

Various genetic mutations of AE1 exchanger proteins have been described, most of the autosomal dominant type.

Hemolytic anemia or hereditary spherocytosis may develop in some patients, accompanied or not by DRTA, since the anion exchanger is also expressed on the red blood cell membrane. The simultaneous presentation of both alterations is frequent in some ethnic groups of South East Asia, The presence of hemolytic anemia depends on the mutation of the gene involved, which is infrequent in the dominant form and frequent in the recessive form of inheritance [18].

The autosomal dominant form of DRTA has a more benign clinical presentation and the manifestations appear in older children, about 5 to 10 years of age; the degree of systemic metabolic acidosis is less severe, with blood bicarbonate values $\cong$ 17 mmol/l and the hypokalemia is less severe or absent. Consequently, the urinary pH is $\geq$6.5. Polyuria in these patients is secondary to a reduction in the maximum capacity of urinary concentration under water restriction, which contributes to the urinary loss of K^+ and hypokalemia. Furthermore, chronic reduction in plasma K^+ concentration contributes to polyuria.

Most of the clinical findings are related to the presence of metabolic acidosis, mainly with failure to thrive and rickets. However, some patients may develop kidney stones and nephrocalcinosis, with progressive loss of renal function, which in most cases may be avoided by early and adequate treatment [8, 19–21].

Chromosomal mutations of the AE1 antiporter, showing as DRTA, have a hereditary dominant transmission and the clinical manifestations may be complete or incomplete. The latter is characterized by having an alkaline pH, but the plasma pH and HCO_3^-values remain normal and stable while the patient stays at a normal steady-state physiological condition. However, the maximum urinary hydrogen ions excretion is reduced under bicarbonate loss by an extrarenal route (e.g., diarrhea). In these cases, the urinary pH is not reduced to $\geq$5.3–5.5, even in the presence of systemic metabolic acidosis, or after the induction of acidosis with an acid load of ammonium chloride ($NH_4^+Cl^-$) [22].

Less frequently, AE1 mutations are seen in children with the recessive hereditary pattern, or with mutations of the H^+ATPase transporter protein. Usually, the manifestations appear at an early age in incomplete form. It always appears early in life in complete form.

Hemolytic anemia is frequent and the clinical manifestations are more severe in the recessive form, mainly in the degree of the electrolyte imbalance, severe metabolic acidosis, failure to thrive, and an early appearance of kidney stones and nephrocalcinosis [22, 23].

Chromosomal and Physiological Alterations of the H^+ATPase Transporter Protein

Chromosomal mutations of the vacuolar H^+ATPase transporter protein are expressed in various cells, such as α-intercalated cells, in the renal collecting tubules, macrophages, and osteoclasts.

Hereditary recessive DRTA is due to chromosomal mutations that encode two of the plasma membrane subunits, the α4 subunit of the ATP6V0A4/7q33-34 gene, which encodes the type-a subunit and the b1 subunit of the ATP6V1B1, 2p13 gene, both present in the apical membrane of the α-intercalated cells, whose function is the extraction of H^+ from the cytosol to the tubular lumen.

The recessive type of DRTA is heterogeneous and may affect different ethnic groups, being secondary to mutations in more than one gene [24–27].

This is the most severe form of distal RTA. The complete clinical presentation happens only in young children <5-year-old, whose clinical manifestations are failure to thrive, hyperchloremic metabolic acidosis with a normal anion gap, and urinary pH > 6.5, which is inappropriately alkaline in the presence of systemic metabolic acidosis. There is also anorexia, vomiting, muscle weakness, and polyuria. The latter is secondary to the reduction in serum potassium (hypokalemia), with hypercalciuria, hypocitraturia, rickets, nephrocalcinosis, renal lithiasis, and progressive sensorineural deafness of early or late onset [28, 29].

Deafness is of the progressive sensorineural type, caused by mutations in the gene encoding the B1 subunit of H^+ ATPase (ATP6V1B1) [30–32]. Deafness is explained, in part, by the mutations described in the B1 subunits, also expressed in the ciliary bodies of the inner ear, causing a reduction of the pH in the endolymph and an increase in the size of the endolymphatic sac, which is detectable by magnetic resonance imaging [33, 34].

Chromosomal and Physiological Alterations of the Carbonic Metalloenzyme Anhydrase II (AC II)

Another molecule that has been detected with mutations causing DRTA is the intracellular enzyme AC II. This metalloenzyme has the widest distribution and catalytic activity in the body. It is expressed in both, proximal and distal renal tubules [35]. Mutations in the gene encoding this protein, which is located on chromosome CA2 8q22, is clinically apparent at an early age, often in the neonatal period, as a severe syndrome of autosomal recessive hereditary type of transmission with mixed RTA, distal and proximal, by what in some nomenclatures is called Mixed RTA, or type III. Therefore, it is characterized by alterations in the proximal tubular bicarbonate recovery, in combination with defects in distal mechanisms of acidification. However, mixed or type III RTA is currently classified as a childhood variant of distal RTA. It is associated with osteopetrosis (marble bones) and brain calcifications, in some phenotypes accompanied also by cognitive changes or mental retardation, bone fractures, deafness, craniofacial dysmorphia with prominent forehead and micrognathia. All this is an addition to the usual clinical manifestations of systemic metabolic acidosis that also are present in other types of RTA [36–39]. More than a dozen heterogeneous mutations have been detected, even in the prenatal period. The prenatal diagnosis is achieved by amniocyte culture or biopsy of the chorionic villi [40–42]. It is considered a rare disease, with an incidence of 1:10^6. This type of RTA may appear in various ethnic groups with a wide geographical distribution, although the frequency is higher in Arab countries [43].

Plausible differential diagnoses to consider with this type of hereditary DRTA may be difficult to assess, based solely on the clinical information. However, a simple clinical diagnostic approach may be supported by the fact that mutations of the H^+ATPase vacuolar protein transporter show clinically a characteristic hereditary recessive type with sensorineural deafness, whereas mutations of the AE1 antiporter present with hemolytic anemia. Mutations of the CA II occur with osteopetrosis. This is a clinical approach, but a chromosomal genetic study is necessary to verify the definitive differential diagnosis [42–44].

The incomplete form of DRTA is characterized by an inability to acidify the urine in the presence of systemic acidosis, or when an overload of H^+ is present. Systemic acidosis does not show up under stable physiological conditions and the blood pH and plasma bicarbonate concentrations are normal. However, metabolic acidosis becomes apparent when an extra-renal loss of bicarbonate, or an increased endogenous or exogenous acid load is present. This is due to the tubular inability to acidify the urine. It is frequently accompanied by renal lithiasis or nephrocalcinosis.

Acid-base and electrolyte alterations of incomplete DRTA are hypokalemia, hypocalcemia, hypercalciuria, and hypocitraturia, as well as an alkaline urine pH. Blood gas results are normal under stable physiological clinical conditions. However, when protein intake increases or, during catabolic stress with increasing organic acid load, a systemic metabolic acidosis develops since there is no adequate renal response to excrete the excess of H^+ in the face of acidosis.

As a consequence of intracellular acidosis, urinary calcium excretion increases, and also the proximal tubular reabsorption of citrates. These alterations lead to the development of hypokalemia and the deposition of calcium salts in the renal interstitium. The administration of ammonium chloride ($NH_4^+Cl^-$) confirms the presence of the urinary acidification defect [45].

Pathophysiology of the Most Frequent Complications of RTA Type I

Extracellular AC IV catalyzes the equilibrium reaction (hydration and dehydration) in the renal tubular lumen of the proximal tubule, to convert HCO_3^- to CO_2 and H_2O. The Na^+/HCO_3^- molecule cannot be reabsorbed as such in the apical membrane. This is the reason to split sodium bicarbonate into two molecules through the equilibrium reaction. Both molecules will be reabsorbed by the apical brush border cell of the proximal tubule. Once in the cytosol, intracellular AC II reverses the reaction to form HCO_3^-, which is reabsorbed as sodium bicarbonate through the basolateral membrane, by the action of the N^+/HCO_3^- co-transporter (NBCe1).

The same function is made by the anion exchanger HCO_3^-/Cl^- (AE1) in the α-intercalated cells of the collecting tubule, so that chromosomal mutations of AC II give place to both, distal and proximal RTA [46, 47].

Osteopetrosis is attributed to a functional deficiency of osteoclasts. AC II is presumed to play an important role in cerebrospinal fluid secretion [48, 49]. However, the etiology of the brain calcifications localized in the paraventricular and basal ganglia is unknown. These lesions usually appear after 5 years of age.

Normal bone resorption performed by the osteoclasts is carried out through the secretion of H^+ ions during the acidification process; this happens in the extracellular resorption of the bone *trabeculae*, requiring the action of H^+ATPase. H^+ ions are generated in the cytosol of osteoclasts during the equilibrium reaction by the action of intracellular AC II, which converts H_2O and CO_2 molecules to HCO_3^- and H^+. AC II deficiency reduces bone resorption capacity, with secondary development of osteopetrosis [40, 49].

Failure to thrive is the result of various mechanisms occurring simultaneously. Metabolic acidosis is an important mechanism leading to failure to thrive in children. Once H^+ ions accumulate in the ECF, the physiological buffer systems become activated, consisting of cation exchange between the extracellular fluid (ECF) and the intracellular fluid (ICF), where H^+ moves into the cells in exchange for intracellular K^+ and Ca^{2+} ions, which leave the cytosol moving to the ECF [50].

Chronic K^+ losses may lead to secondary hyperaldosteronism, with persistent hypokalemia characteristic of RTA type I, II, and III. Another factor that stimulates the renin-angiotensin-aldosterone system (RAAS) is the persistent volume reduction of the ECF, caused by anorexia, vomiting, polyuria, and dehydration. All this aggravates chronic K^+ depletion and also contributes to the development of failure to thrive [51].

Children with DRTA develop polyuria secondary to renal losses of bicarbonate, as well as Na^+, K^+, phosphates, citrates, and magnesium. Renal losses of Na^+ and H_2O favor the contraction of the ECF volume and activation of the RAAS, which increases the urinary K^+ losses. Chronic metabolic acidosis and hypokalemia contribute together to the development of failure to thrive [48].

The calcium bone losses during the buffering mechanism of metabolic acidosis lead also to the development of rickets, if untreated. The highest concentration of calcium in the body is found in bone, where Ca^{2+} binds to phosphate molecules to form deposits of hydroxyapatite [52]. Therefore, metabolic acidosis is associated with an increase in urinary calcium excretion leading to bone demineralization and the onset of rickets. Increased bone resorption occurs through various mechanisms. In cases of chronic metabolic acidosis, the reduction of the systemic pH and the reduction of the plasma HCO_3^- increase osteoclastic activity, thus, the resorption of Ca^{2+} from the bone.

Another mechanism of calcium extraction from bone, in cases of metabolic acidosis, includes the cyclo-oxygenase system with the release of prostaglandin PGE_2. These prostaglandins stimulate the expression of the nuclear activator receptor κ-B (RANK) and H^+ATPase, both capable of stimulating osteoclast activity [53].

In addition to urinary calcium losses, there is a reduction of intestinal calcium absorption, due to alterations of the enzymatic hydroxylation of 25-hydroxyvitamin-D and its conversion to 1, 25-dihydroxyvitamin-D. This was found in rats after an oral administration of ammonium chloride ($NH_4^+Cl^-$). Correcting the metabolic acidosis will revert the calcium metabolism alterations to the normal state [35].

A reduction in the secretion of growth hormone (GH) and insulin-like growth factor (IGF-1) has also been implicated as mechanisms of failure to thrive and rickets since metabolic acidosis tends to diminish growth hormone and IGF-1 action in the bone's growth plates [54].

Chronic metabolic acidosis favors the development of renal nephrocalcinosis and lithiasis by different mechanisms that alter calcium physiology.

Failure to thrive and rickets are also caused by the suppression of the activity of the calcium sensor-receptor (CaSR) by metabolic acidosis, since it affects the physiological control of the parathyroid hormone, with further deterioration of the systemic and renal metabolism of calcium [55].

Patients with DRTA have an alkaline urinary pH, hypercalciuria, and with some frequency, hypocitraturia. This combination of factors is of high risk for the development of renal nephrocalcinosis and lithiasis, which, in turn, lead to chronic renal failure and secondary hyperparathyroidism, especially in patients with a late diagnosis or inadequate treatment, which worsens in cases with recurrent urinary tract infections [56, 57].

Precipitation and formation of calcium/phosphate salt deposits depend on numerous factors that promote or inhibit the crystallization process, such as extracellular, intracellular, and intraluminal tubular pH; the ionic concentration of calcium and phosphates, as well as the reduction of crystallization inhibitors, such as citrates, sulfates, pyrophosphates, magnesium, glycosaminoglycans, and nephrocalcin, among others.

Patients with DRTA have a high urinary pH (≥ 6.5) and a reduced water load to the distal tubule, facilitating the development of calcifications of the renal medullary area (nephrocalcinosis) or the renal tubular lumen (nephrolithiasis) [58]. In proximal RTA (type II), this complication is rare, although most calcium and oxalates are reabsorbed in the proximal tubule. However, this tubular area is protected by the presence of aquaporins that provide abundant H_2O, which is reabsorbed by the cells of the brush border. Furthermore, the intracellular pH is reduced, favoring the reabsorption of citrates and other salts, such as magnesium and sulfates, which reduce the precipitation of calcium oxalate salts.

On the contrary, in DRTA (type I) the amount of water is diminished by the reduction of the ECF volume, as well as by the repeated episodes of systemic dehydration in children with this entity [59, 60]. Intracellular pH increases the reabsorption of citrates at the proximal tubular area, reducing the distal load (hypocitraturia). This increases the distal tubular precipitation of calcium salts. Hypocitraturia, together with the reduction of H_2O intake, is a common denominator of the development of lithiasis and nephrocalcinosis in diverse pathological conditions [60].

Diagnosis and Treatment of DRTA in Pediatric Patients

First, it is a priority to diagnose the presence of systemic metabolic acidosis. Otherwise, reaching the diagnosis of any type of RTA will be out of the question. This is the main feature for over-diagnosing RTA in Mexico and some other Latin American countries, during the last few years [61].

The four types of RTA described so far have hyperchloremic metabolic acidosis, with normal anion gap and, persistent alkaline urinary pH (due to renal tubular defects of HCO_3^- reabsorption), and retention of H^+, mainly as NH_4^+. The differential diagnosis of primary or secondary DRTA, as well as with other types of RTA, is based on the study of the renal capacity to acidify the urine. The laboratory studies must include the determination of arterial blood gases or from arterialized venous blood (without the application of a tourniquet), urinary anion gap, ammonium excretion, the difference of the partial pressure of carbon dioxide in blood and urine (pCO_2 U/P), by the use of urine acidification stimulation tests. It is important to take into account the age of the patient to make an accurate interpretation of the blood gas results. The diagnosis of systemic metabolic acidosis in children should be done by using as a reference the normal laboratory values according to the child's age. The use of normal adult values as a reference for children ought to be avoided. The details of the diagnostic tools for diagnosing RTA are discussed in other publications [61, 62], as well as herein in Chap. 7.

Treatment of DRTA needs a multidisciplinary approach, including the management of the etiology, such as the suspension of nephrotoxic drugs, or the treatment of the immune disease that causes the secondary RTA.

In the case of primary or hereditary DRTA, there is no specific treatment, thus, the management of the complications of acid-base and electrolyte imbalance should be carried out accordingly. Special attention should be paid to the management and treatment of failure to thrive, avoiding at the same time the development of nephrocalcinosis and nephrolithiasis. This will prevent damage to the renal parenchyma and further progression to end-stage kidney disease (ESKD).

Therefore, the therapeutic objective is to correct hypokalemia, hypocitraturia, hypercalciuria, and hypophosphatemia, a priority measure to improve growth, avoiding the development of nephrocalcinosis [63].

Firstly, it is of utmost importance to correct the potassium deficiency at an early stage of treatment, when severe hypokalemia is present and, proceed to correct the acidosis afterward, since the administration of alkalinizing solutions facilitates K^+ ions shifting into the ICF, worsening the hypokalemia [62].

Once the hypokalemia has been corrected, a dose of alkaline solutions containing bicarbonate is recommended, 1–3 mEq/kg/day, requiring dose adjustments until the hypercalciuria and hypocitraturia decrease back to normal. The total dose is divided into three or four daily doses; the administration of a higher nightly dose is recommended.

Citrate is useful in the presence of combined hypocitraturia and hypercalciuria. Potassium citrate is preferred over sodium citrate since the latter favors hypercalciuria. Citrate is converted to bicarbonate in the liver after entering the Krebs cycle. Urine alkalinization reduces citrate reabsorption, increasing citrates distal load, and favors the solubility of cystine, calcium oxalate, and uric acid. This helps to reduce the risk of nephrolithiasis and nephrocalcinosis. However, care should be taken not to alkalinize the urinary pH excessively, because it can favor the precipitation of calcium phosphates [63]. The chemical composition of different alkalizing solutions available in the market.

The prognosis is favorable when the diagnosis is made early and the therapeutic measures are instituted expeditiously. Electrolyte and acid-base metabolism disturbances, as well as failure to thrive, are corrected with the alkalizing treatment. Furthermore, nephrocalcinosis and nephrolithiasis are avoided or minimized with appropriate and early treatment.

References

1. Lightwood R. Calcium infarction of the kidneys in infants. Arch Dis Child. 1935;10:205–6.
2. Rodriguez Soriano J. Renal tubular acidosis: the clinical entity. J Am Soc Nephrol. 2002;13(8):2160–70.
3. Morris RC Jr, Fudenberg HH. Impaired renal acidification in patients with hypergammaglobulinemia. Medicine. 1967;46:57–69N.
4. Talal N. Sjogren's syndrome, lymphoproliferation and, renal tubular acidosis. Ann Intern Med. 1971;74:633–4.
5. DuBose TD, Good DW, Hamm LL, Wall SM. Ammonium transport in the kidney: new physiological concepts and their clinical implications. J Am Soc Nephrol. 1991;1:1193–203.
6. Alper SL, Natale J, Gluck S, et al. Subtypes of intercalated cells in rat kidney collecting duct defined by antibodies against erythroid band 3 and renal vacuolar H^+-ATPase. Proc Natl Acad Sci U S A. 1989;86:5429–33.
7. Wall SM, Fischer MP. Contribution of the Na(+)-K(+)-2Cl(−) cotransporter (NKCC1) to transepithelial transport of H(+), NH(4)(+), K(+), and Na(+) in rat outer medullary collecting duct. Am Soc Nephrol. 2002;13(4):827–35.
8. Darman RB, Chernova MN, et al. The AE gene family of $Cl/HCO3^-$ exchangers. J Nephrol. 2002;15(Suppl 5):S41–53.
9. Halperin ML, Kamel KS, Goldstein MB: Principles of acid-base physiology. En Halperin ML, Kamel KS, Goldstein MB (eds): Fluid, electrolyte, and acid-base physiology 4th ed. Saunders Elsevier, Philadelphia, 2010: 3-28.
10. Dobyan DC, Bulger RE. Renal carbonic anhydrase. Am J Phys. 1982;243(4):F311–24S.
11. Endeward V, Cartron JP, Ripoche P, Gros G. RhAG protein of the Rhesus complex is a CO2 channel in the human red cell membrane. FASEB J. 2008;22:64–73.
12. Carrisoza-Gaytan R, Rangel C, Salvador C, Saldaña-Meyer R, Escalona C, Satlin LM, Liu W, Zavilowitz B, Joyce Trujillo J, Bobadilla NA, Escobar LI. The hyperpolarization-activated cyclic nucleotide-gated HCN2 channel transports ammonium in the distal nephron. Kidney Int. 2011;80:832–40. https://doi.org/10.1038/ki.2011.230.
13. Weiner ID, Hamm LL. Molecular mechanisms of renal ammonia transport. Annu Rev Physiol. 2007;69:317–40.
14. Escobar L, Mejía N, Gil H, Gil H, Santos F, Santos F. La acidosis tubular renal distal: una enfermedad hereditaria en la que no se pueden eliminar los hidrogeniones. Nefrologia. 2013;33(3):289–96.

15. Battle D, Haque SK. Genetic causes and mechanisms of distal renal tubular acidosis. Nephrol Dial Transplant. 2012;10:3691–704.
16. Chial H. Mendelian genetics: patterns of inheritance and single-gene disorders. Nat Educat. 2008;1(1):63.
17. Alper SL. Molecular physiology and genetics of Na^{+}-independent SLC4 anion. Exp Biol. 2009;212:1672–83.
18. Wagner S, Vogel R, Lietzke R, et al. Immunochemical characterization of a band 3-like anion exchanger in collecting duct of the human kidney. Am J Phys. 1987;253:F213–21.
19. Jarolim P, Shayakul C, Prabakaran D, et al. Autosomal dominant distal renal tubular acidosis is associated in three families with heterozygosity for the R589H mutation in the AE1 (band 3) Cl^{-}/HCO3− exchanger. J Biol Chem. 1998;273:638–6388.
20. Karet FE, Gainza FJ, Györy AZ, Unwin RJ, Wrong O, Tanner MJ, et al. Mutations in the chloride-bicarbonate exchanger gene AE1 cause autosomal dominant but not autosomal recessive distal renal tubular acidosis. Proc Natl Acad Sci. 1998;95:6337–42.
21. Bruce LJ, Cope DL, Jones GK, Schofield AE, Burley M, Povey S, et al. Familial distal renal tubular acidosis is associated with mutations in the red cell anion exchanger (Band 3, AE1) gene. J Clin Invest. 1997;100:693–707, 56.
22. Battle D, Ghanekar H, Jain S, et al. Hereditary distal renal tubular acidosis: new understandings. Ann Rev Med. 2001;52:471–84.
23. Alper SL. Familial renal tubular acidosis. J Nephrol. 2010;23(Suppl 16):S57–76.
24. Garg LC. Respective roles of H-ATPase and H-K-ATPase in ion transport in the kidney. J Am Soc Nephrol. 1991;2(5):949–60.
25. Blake-Palmer KG, Karet FE. Cellular physiology of the renal H_ATPase. Curr Opin Nephrol Hypertens. 2009;18:433–8.
26. Schuster VL. Function and regulation of collecting duct intercalated cells. Annu Rev Physiol. 1993;55:267–88.
27. Karet FE, Finberg KE, Nelson RD, Nayir A, Mocan H, Sanjad SA, et al. Mutations in the gene encoding B1 subunit of H -ATPase cause renal tubular acidosis with sensorineural deafness. Nat Genet 1999;21:84–90; Karet FE. Inherited distal renal tubular acidosis. J Am Soc Nephrol. 2002;13:2178–84.
28. Vargas-Poussou R, Houillier P, Le Pottier N, Strompf L, Loirat C, Baudouin V, et al. Genetic investigation of autosomal recessive distal renal tubular acidosis: evidence for early sensorineural hearing loss associated with mutations in the ATP6V0A4 gene. J Am Soc Nephrol. 2006;17:1437–43.
29. Stover EH, Borthwick KJ, Bavalia C, Eady N, Fritz DM, Rungroj N, et al. Novel ATP6V1B1 and ATP6V0A4 mutations in autosomal recessive distal renal tubular acidosis with new evidence for hearing loss. J Med Genet. 2002;39:796–803, 63.
30. Santos F, Rey C, Málaga S, Rodríguez LM, Orejas G. The syndrome of renal tubular acidosis and nerve deafness. Discordant manifestations in dizygotic twin brothers. Pediatr Nephrol. 1991;5:2357.
31. Miura K, Sekine T, Takahashi K, Takita J, Harita Y, Ohki K, et al. Mutational analyses of the ATP6V1B1 and ATP6V0A4 genes in patients with primary distal renal tubular acidosis. Nephrol Dial Transplant. 2013;28:2123–30.
32. Nishi T, Forgac M. The vacuolar (H^{+})-ATPases-nature's most versatile proton pumps. Nat Rev Mol Cell Biol. 2002;3:94–103.
33. Rink N, Bitzan M, O'Gorman G, et al. Endolymphatic sac enlargement in a girl with a novel mutation for distal renal tubular acidosis and severe deafness. Case Rep Pediatr. 2012;2012:605–53.
34. Goodman AD, Lemann J, Lennon EJ. Production, excretion and, a net balance of fixed acid in patients with renal acidosis. J Clin Invest. 1965;44:495–506.
35. Baird TT, Waheed A, Okuyama T, et al. Catalysis and inhibition of human carbonic anhydrase IV. Biochemistry. 1997;36:2669–78.

36. Battle D, Ghanekar H, Jain S, et al. Hereditary distal renal tubular acidosis: a new understanding. Annu Rev Med. 2001;52:471–4.
37. Schwartz GJ. Physiology and molecular biology of renal carbonic anhydrase. J Nephrol. 2002;15(Suppl 5):S61–74.
38. Purkerson JM, Schwartz GJ. The role of carbonic anhydrases in renal physiology. Kidney Int. 2007;71:103–15.
39. Shah GN, Bonapace G, Hu PY, Strisciuglio P, Sly WS. Carbonic anhydrase II deficiency syndrome (osteopetrosis with renal tubular acidosis and brain calcification): novel mutations in CA2 identified by direct sequencing expand the opportunity for genotype-phenotype correlation. Hum Mutat. 2004;24(3):272; Sly WS, Sato S, Zhu XL. Evaluation of carbonic anhydrase isozymes in disorders involving osteopetrosis and/or renal tubular acidosis. Clin Biochem. 1991;4:311–8.
40. Marks SC Jr. Morphological evidence of reduced bone resorption in osteopetrotic (op) mice. Am J Anat. 1982;163:157–67.
41. Strisciuglio P, Sartorio R, Pecoraro C, Lotito F, Sly WS. Variable clinical presentation of carbonic anhydrase deficiency: evidence for heterogeneity? Eur J Pediatr. 1990;149:337–40.
42. Hu PY, Roth DE, Skaggs LA, Venta PJ, Tashian RE, Guibaud P, et al. A splice junction mutation in intron 2 of the carbonic anhydrase II gene of osteopetrosis patients from Arabic countries. Hum Mutat. 1992;1:288–92.
43. Sly WS, Hewett-Emmett D, Whyte MP, Yu YS, Tashian RE. Carbonic anhydrase II deficiency is identified as the primary defect in the autosomal recessive syndrome of osteopetrosis with renal tubular acidosis and cerebral calcification. Proc Natl Acad Sci U S A. 1983;80(9):2752–6.
44. Choi JS, Kim CS, Park JW, Bae EH, Ma SK, Kim SW. Incomplete distal renal tubular acidosis with nephrocalcinosis. Chonnam Med J. 2011;47(3):170–2. https://doi.org/10.4068/cmj.2011.47.3.170. Epub 2011 Dec 26. PMID: 22247918.
45. Soleimani M. $Na^{+}HCO_3$ cotransporter (NBC): expression and regulation in the kidney. J Nephrol. 2002;15(Suppl 5):S32–40.
46. Herrin JT. Renal tubular acidosis. In: Avner ED, Harmon WE, Niaudet P, editors. Pediatric nephrology. 5th ed. Philadelphia: Lippincott Williams & Wilkins; 2004. p. 757–76.
47. Bushinsky DA, Frick KK. The effects of acid on bone. Curr Opin Nephrol Hypertens. 2000;9:369–79.
48. Blair HC, Teitelbaum SL, Ghiselli R, et al. Osteoclastic bone resorption by a polarized vacuolar proton pump. Science. 1989;245:855–7.
49. Halperin ML, Kamel KS, Goldstein MB. Potassium physiology. In: Halperin ML, Kamel KS, Goldstein MB, editors. Fluid, electrolyte, and acid-base physiology. 4th ed. Philadelphia: Saunders Elsevier; 2010. p. 425–59.
50. Fry AC, Karet FE. Inherited renal acidoses. Physiology (Bethesda). 2007;22:202–11.
51. Bushinsky DA. Stimulated osteoclastic and suppressed osteoblastic activity in metabolic but not respiratory acidosis. Am J Phys. 1995;268:C80–8.
52. Frick KK, Bushinsky DA. Metabolic acidosis stimulates RANKL RNA expression in bone through a cyclo-oxygenase-dependent mechanism. J Bone Miner Res. 2003;18:1317–25.
53. Chan JCM, Oldham SB. DeLuca HF, an effectiveness of 1-alpha-hydroxyvitamin D3 in children with renal osteodystrophy associated with hemolysis. J Pediatr. 1977;90:820–4.
54. Campion KL, McCormick WD, Warwicker J, Bin Khayat ME, Atkinson-Dell RC, Delbridge LW, Mun H-C, Conigrave AD, Ward DT. Pathophysiologic changes in extracellular pH modulate parathyroid calcium-sensing receptor activity and secretion *via* a histidine-independent mechanism. J Am Soc Nephrol. 2015;9:2163–71. https://doi.org/10.1681/ASN.2014070653.
55. Velázquez JL. Acidosis tubular renal. Bol Med Hosp Infant Mex. 2012;69:502–8.
56. Alexander RT, Cordat E, Chambrey R, Dimke H, Eladari D. Acidosis and urinary calcium excretion: insights from genetic disorders. Am Soc Nephrol. 2016;27(12):3511–20.
57. Guerra-Hernández NE, Ordaz-López KV, Escobar-Pérez L, Gómez-Tenorio C, García-Nieto VM. Distal renal tubular acidosis screening by urinary acidification testing in Mexican children. Rev Investig Clin. 2015;67(3):191–8.

58. Milliner DS. Urolithiasis. In: Avner ED, Harmon WE, Niaudet P, editors. Pediatric nephrology. 5th ed. Philadelphia: Lippincott Williams & Wilkins; 2004. p. 1191–11.
59. Sikora P, Roth B, Kribs A, Michalk DV, Hesse A. Hoppe B Hypocitraturia is one of the major risk factors for nephrocalcinosis in very low birth weight (VLBW) infants. Kidney Int. 2003 Jun;63(6):2194–9.
60. Muñoz AR, Escobar L, Medeiros DM. Sobre-diagnóstico de acidosis tubular renal en México. Rev Investig Clin. 2012;4(64):399–401.
61. García Nieto V, Rodrigo Jiménez MD. Pruebas de función tubular. Tubulopatías. Nefrología. 2012;7. https://doi.org/10.3265/Nefrologia.2010.pub1.ed80.chapter2794.
62. Muñoz AR, Escobar L, Medeiros DM. Acidosis tubular renal en niños: conceptos actuales de diagnóstico y tratamiento. Bol Med Hosp Infant Mex. 2013;70:1665–146.
63. Morris RC Jr, Sebastian A. Alkali therapy in renal tubular acidosis: who needs it? J Am Soc Nephrol. 2002;13:2186–8.

Chapter 10
Hyperkalemic Renal Tubular Acidosis (RTA Type IV)

Jesús Lagunas-Muñoz and Ricardo Muñoz

Introduction

Four types of renal tubular acidosis (ATR) are defined. RTA Types I, II, and III are described in the corresponding chapters of this work. Contrary to what happens in adulthood, Type IV RTA with hyperkalemia is the least frequent type of RTA in children; laboratory findings show a systemic metabolic acidosis, with increased blood potassium concentration [K^+] and normal anion gap.

RTA Type IV originates either from a deficit in production or a reduction in aldosterone activity (hypoaldosteronism). Also, it may be due to a lack of renal tubular response to aldosterone ("pseudo-hypoaldosteronism"). Aldosterone is produced in the *zona glomerulosa* of the adrenal cortex; its main function is Na^+ reabsorption and increased activity of the Na^+ reabsorption channels (ENaC) upon the apical

J. Lagunas-Muñoz (✉)
Department of Pediatric Nephrology, National Medical Center La Raza, Mexican Institute of Social Security, Mexico City, Mexico

High Specialty Medical Unit, General Hospital "Dr. Gaudencio González Garza." National Medical Center La Raza, Mexican Institute of Social Security, Mexico City, Mexico

R. Muñoz
Retired from: Department of Pediatric Nephrology, Hemodialysis Unit, The Children's Hospital at Albany Medical Center, Albany, NY, USA

Retired from: Pediatric Nephrology Department, Hospital Infantil de México Federico Gómez, Mexico City, Mexico

Retired from: Research Division, Hospital Infantil de Mexico Federico Gomez, Mexico City, Mexico

Retired from: National System of Investigators, Level I, Mexico City, Mexico

Retired from: North American Pediatric Renal Transplantation Collaborative Study (NAPRTCS) Study, Woburn, MA, USA

R. Muñoz (ed.), *Renal Tubular Acidosis in Children*,
https://doi.org/10.1007/978-3-030-91940-5_10

membrane of the principal cells of the distal tubules, at the "Aldosterone Sensitive Zone", as well as K^+ secretion at the principal cells of the distal nephron (connecting and collecting tubules).

Type IV RTA is a distal nephron alteration. However, the kidneys do not lose the ability to acidify the urine, so the urine pH can be reduced to ≤ 5.5, because the H^+ATPase transporter protein, located in the α-intercalated cells of the collecting tubule, is intact and displays a normal function [1].

Physiological Mechanisms and Renal Pathophysiology in RTA with Hyperkalemia

The mechanisms of systemic and renal physiology, as well as the pathology of K^+ metabolism, are described in more detail in Chaps. 2 and 3 of this publication.

In this chapter, the information is aimed at describing some of the physiological mechanisms and the clinical manifestations specifically present in the pediatric age group, compared to the adult population. Also, the main clinical entities that may be associated with a hyperkalemic Type IV RTA in children will be described herein.

As described in the previous chapters, the greatest amount of bicarbonate and potassium filtered in the glomeruli are reabsorbed at the proximal tubules. The same is true for K^+ and H^+, but the highest secretion of these ions occurs at the distal level of the nephron, where H^+ ions are exchanged for bicarbonate during this process.

The finest regulation of fluids and electrolytes, as well as of acid-base metabolism, takes place in the distal nephron, where the principal cells and the α- and β-intercalated cells perform these functions. The α- and β-intercalated cells are located in the connecting and collecting tubules; they comprise ~30% of the cells in the distal nephron. The apical membrane of these cells is the site of the H^+-adenosine-triphosphatase pump (H^+ATPase), also called H^+ATPase vacuolar (VH^+ATPase), is expressed. This H^+ ion transporter protein is responsible for H^+ secretion and, consequently, the acidification of the urine. Secondarily to this process, new bicarbonate is formed (Fig. 10.1).

H^+ATPase, an electrogenic pump, transports protons (H^+ ions) from the cytoplasm to the tubular lumen through the apical membrane.

Once protons are excreted into the tubular lumen, excretion in the final urine is carried out by different physiological mechanisms. One consists of the excretion of free H^+, which is only a small amount of the total H^+ ions excreted. Nonetheless, excretion of free H^+ is important, since it determines the urinary pH, a marker used to determine the renal capacity to acidify the urine.

The main bulk of H^+ is excreted in the collecting tubule as NH_3/NH_4^+ (ammonia/ammonium) buffer solution, plus weak phosphoric acids ($HPO_4^=/H_2PO_4^-$) and sulfuric ($HSO_4^=/H_2SO_4^-$), whose combined renal excretion is called titratable acidity.

K^+ secretion is carried out mainly by the proton/potassium pump H^+K^+ATPase, which exchanges K^+ for H^+ in the apical membrane of the α-intercalated cells of the

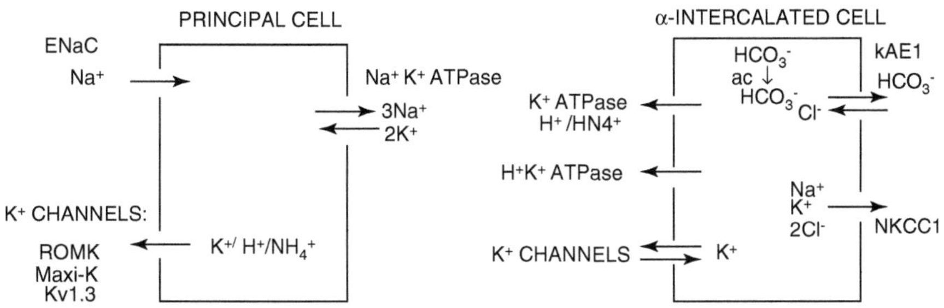

Fig. 10.1 Diagram of the functions of the principal and α-intercalated cell in the cortical collecting tubule. The principal cell reabsorbs Na^+ from the tubular lumen in the apical membrane through sodium channels (ENaC) and from the interstitium through the basolateral membrane by Na^+K^+ATPase in exchange for K^+, which is secreted into the tubular lumen through the apical K^+ channels: ROMK and others. A transtubular electronegative gradient is generated, which facilitates Na^+ reabsorption and K^+ secretion in a continuous cycle. The highest H^+ excretion is carried out in the α-intercalated cells via the transporter molecules H^+ATPase and H^+K^+ATPase, for its final excretion as NH_4^+ and titratable acidity. As a consequence of H^+ excretion, new HCO_3- is formed from intracellular CO_2 and H_2O, in the presence of carbonic anhydrase II (ac). The bicarbonate is reabsorbed through the basolateral membrane by the exchanger AE1, in exchange for Cl^-. The KCl-KCC4 cotransporter is expressed in the basolateral membrane, maintaining low levels of chloride in the intracellular space

so-called "distal nephron sensitive to aldosterone" (DNSA), whose effectiveness is increased by the Na^+K^+ATPase in the basolateral membrane. This protein exchanger extracts Na^+ from the cytosol to the interstitium in exchange for K^+. In turn, the accumulated intracellular K^+ is excreted from the cell into the tubular lumen by H^+K^+ATPase, closing the cycle. The negative transepithelial voltage acquired by this mechanism increases, improving the never-ending cycle of Na^+ tubular reabsorption [2–4].

The principal cells make up the remaining ~70% of the functional cells in the distal nephron. In the luminal (apical) membrane of the principal cells are located the epithelial sodium channels (ENaC), as well as the amiloride-sensitive Na^+/Cl^+ (NCC) channels (Fig. 10.1). Besides, these channels can be blocked by other drugs, such as triamterene, pentamidine, and trimethoprim [4–7]. The Na^+/K^+ATPase transporter protein is located in the basolateral membrane of the principal cell. It is an energy-dependent primary active transport system. Its function consists of the reabsorption of 3 Na^+ molecules in exchange for 2 K^+ molecules, the latter coming from the interstitium (peritubular fluid). Na^+/K^+ATPase regulates Na^+Cl^- reabsorption in the renal tubules. The intracellular/extracellular transepithelial potential difference (−60 mV intracellular), originated from the high concentration of intracellular potassium [K^+], and the reabsorption of Na^+, favors continuous reabsorption of Na^+ from the lumen into the cytoplasm, and to the extracellular fluid (ECF) [7–9]. The use of cyclosporine interferes with the sodium gradient in the collecting duct cells and blocks Na^+K^+ATPase, as well as the K^+ channels described next [10].

Table 10.1 Factors that determine the renal tubular excretion of potassium [14]

Trans-tubular K^+ gradient (principal cell, apical membrane):
GTTK
Aldosterone bioactivity
K^+ channels permeability
Distal tubular urine flow
Na^+ distal tubular load
Degree of electronegativity of the renal tubular lumen generated by Na^+ reabsorption in the ENaC and Na^+ Cl channels
Composition and concentration of urinary anions

The apical membranes of the principal cells of the connecting and collecting tubules are located in the external renal medulla, where they express the rectifying potassium channels, ROMK ("renal outer medullary small conductance K^+ channels"), whose function is the secretion of potassium from the cytosol into the tubular lumen [6]. A similar function is played by other channels that regulate K^+ secretion, such as the K^+Cl^- cotransporter (KCC), located in the basolateral membrane and the BK channels, also called maxi K^+, among others, described in recent years and are relevant in the excretion and renal handling of K^+ [11–13].

Principal cells also contribute, though indirectly, to the secretion of H^+, as a result of sodium transport via ENaC, which generates the electronegative gradient that favors the secretion of H^+ and K^+ through the transporter proteins H^+ATPase and H^+K^+ ATPase, located in the apical membrane of the α-intercalated cells. The reduction of the transepithelial voltage reduces the secretion of both ions.

The reabsorption of Na^+, and the secretion and excretion of K^+ are finely regulated by aldosterone and other important factors, mentioned in Table 10.1.

Aldosterone is a hormone with multiple functions, produced mainly in the *zona glomerulosa* of the adrenal cortex in reciprocal regulation of the renin-angiotensin-aldosterone system (RAAS), preferentially with angiotensin II (Ag II). It participates in specific functions of the cardiovascular system (arteriolar and endothelial), and at the renal tubular level in Na^+ reabsorption and K^+ and H^+ excretion. Thus, aldosterone is a determining factor in maintaining the volume and composition of body fluids and blood pressure. Also, aldosterone participates in the regulation of acid-base metabolism in different ways [15].

Aldosterone has a moderate activity on Na^+K^+ATPase at a systemic level. The main target organ of the hormone is the principal cells of the distal nephron (NDSA) that comprises the final part of the distal convoluted tubule, connecting tubule, and cortical collecting tubule.

Aldosterone binds to its mineralocorticoid receptor (MR) that transfer aldosterone to the cell nucleus, where it activates the transcription of several genes, including the gene encoding the glucocorticoid regulatory kinase 1 (SGK1), which stimulates the production of ENaC, Na^+K^+ATPase, and the apical rectifying channels ROMK [16]. This increases the renal tubular reabsorption of Na^+, thus the depolarization of the apical membrane creating a negative luminal transepithelial electrical potential, which in turn favors the secretion of K^+ by the principal cells. Likewise, in an independent mechanism of Na^+ reabsorption and K^+ secretion, aldosterone stimulates the secretion of H^+ in the α-intercalated cells, facilitating urinary acidification by increasing H^+ ATPase at the apical membrane of the collecting tubule [17–23].

The α-subunit of the Na^+/K^+ATPase is the physiologically active part of this protein, and confers the highest activity to the Na^+K^+ATPase molecule [24]. Its production is reduced in newborn infants of different mammalian species, compared to that in adults of the same species. This has been demonstrated in tissues of various organs and different segments of the nephron [24].

At the systemic level, the largest amount of total Na^+ is distributed within the ECF, while K^+ is mostly restricted to the ICF (intracellular fluid) by the Na^+K^+ATPase antiporter, keeping sodium out and potassium inside the cell, a mechanism favored by the presence of insulin and catecholamines and, to a lesser extent by aldosterone, glucagon, growth hormone, thyroid hormone, and physical exercise, which facilitate the entry of K^+ into the cell, thus preventing the accumulation of this ion in the ECF, at a time when a significant increase of K^+ ensues [25].

The volume of the body fluids depends on the total amount of electrolytes retained in each space, which, in turn, retains a proportional amount of water. Since sodium is the most abundant electrolyte in the ECF, the volume is determined by the amount of total Na^+ and water retained in such fluid space. Water is retained in the ECF in a proportion of 1000 ml H_2O/154 mEq of Na^+.

On the other hand, the amount of total K^+ determines the volume of the ICF. This is in terms of the regulation of the volume of the body fluid compartments, which is done by regulating the volume of each cell in the body. Thus, the total amount of Na^+ and K^+ regulates the volume, not the osmolality of the body fluids.

On the other hand, the total amount of H_2O regulates the osmolality of the fluid spaces. Therefore, a bigger amount of H_2O renders a more diluted solution, meaning the solutes (electrolytes and other water-soluble particles) become less concentrated in such a solution (hypoosmolality). On the contrary, the less amount of water, the more concentrated the solution is, and the solutes are more concentrated (hyperosmolality).

Based on the above physiological concepts, there are important differences between the osmolality and electrolyte values found in children, compared to adults.

In adults, total body water (TBW) is the equivalent of ≅ 55–60% of the body weight, while the ECF and ICF volume compartments are about the same size.

In the pediatric age, on the other hand, the TBW is 60–65% of the body weight (according to the age); about 80% in the newborn and 80–90% in the premature (according to the degree of prematurity). The reason for the increase in the amount of total body water in children occurs at the expense of the physiological increased size of the ECF during the pediatric-age period [26].

The concentration of Na^+ in the ECF measured in blood $[Na^+]$s is 135–145 mmol/l in the adult, but when measured by ultracentrifuge in the water of the ECF, it is 154 mmol/l, which provides an osmolality of 285 ± 5 mOsm/kg H_2O.

The lowest K^+ concentration [K^+] is in the ECF, with blood values of 3.5–5.2 mmol/l, while in the ICF is 140–160 mmol/l.

On the other hand, in the pediatric age group [Na^+]p in the ECF is 130–140 mmol/l and 7–15 mmol/l in the ICF, which provides an osmolality of 280 ± 5 mOsm/kg H_2O. In the child [K^+]s is 3.0–6.0 mmol/l, depending on the age. There is an inverse relationship between gestational age and [K^+]s; thus, at a lower gestational age [K^+]s is higher [27, 28].

The figures shown herein are just some examples of the physiological differences between the pediatric age versus adulthood, which is why the interpretation of the findings of acid-base and electrolyte metabolism based on the normal values in adults renders completely undesirable and should be avoided.

These physiological differences in the volume of the body fluids between adults and children have an impact on the renal physiology of electrolytes and acid-base metabolism at different ages.

Perhaps, the reduction of the activity of the α-subunit of the transporter Na^+K^+ATPase exchanger in children may play a role in the marked differences present in the ECF volume increase, as compared to the ICF. This concept is compatible with increased renal sodium losses related to the filtered load, which is manifested clinically by an increased fractional Na^+ excretion (FENa). Also, it may explain the [K^+] reduction of the ICF and an increase of [K^+] in the ECF, as it has been measured in muscle tissues of newborn and premature animals.

Thus, it may be feasible that in children, the reduction of the activity of the α-subunit of Na^+K^+ATPase is related to the marked differences in the increased volume of the ECF compared to the ECF, and also with the reduction of [K^+] in the ICF and the increase of [K^+] in the ECF, as measured in muscle tissues of newborn and premature animals. Increased ECF volume should be linked to total Na^+ body retention. However, the fractional excretion of the filtered Na^+ (FENa) is very high in the premature (5–6%) and the newborn (2–3%), decreasing progressively during the first years of life, while in the adult it is $\leq$1%.

Moreover, there is a physiological increased excretion of glucose, albumin, citrates, urates, bicarbonate, amino acids, etc., in the newborn period, perhaps because the tubular reabsorption of these substances is coupled to the tubular handling of sodium, as a consequence of the reduction of Na^+K^+ATPase in the pediatric age group [29].

However, in premature babies, newborns, and early in life, the excretion of K^+ is reduced, although the concentration of aldosterone runs high. In theory, the reduction of the Na^+ K^+ATPase activity plays a role in this mechanism [30]. Na^+K^+ATPase is almost non-existent in the fetus and its production increase about four-fold or more at birth. During weaning, it rises again and continues to increase progressively throughout the pediatric age period [31].

Acid-base regulation and body potassium metabolism are intertwined; alterations in one component modify the other in two ways, at the systemic level and, specifically in renal tubular reabsorption and excretion of K^+ and H^+. The increase in [K^+]s stimulates urinary potassium excretion and decreases ammonium synthesis, while K^+ depletion leads to the opposite effect.

Human studies and the results of experimental interventions carried out to date in animals, mainly in rats and dogs, are controversial. Hyperkalemia inhibits the production of ammonia in the proximal tubules. However, contrary to what happens in experimental animal studies, in humans with hyperkalemia the final excretion of NH_4^+ is not reduced despite the reduction of ammonium production, perhaps due to the important role in H^+ regulation in the distal nephron. The increase in $[K^+]s$ is one of the factors that stimulates aldosterone secretion, which in turn, results in increased distal renal tubular secretion of K^+ and H^+. Furthermore, the increase in Na^+ reabsorption and K^+ secretion in the principal cells stimulate ammonium synthesis, which occurs along the nephron, but mainly in the mitochondria of the brush border cells of the proximal tubule. Although hyperkalemia reduces the production of ammonium, aldosterone compensates for this effect with an increase in the distal tubular load and secretion of NH_3/NH_4^+ in α-intercalated cells. Therefore, aldosterone contributes indirectly to the urinary acidification process [32].

Hyperkalemia is the result of a reduction in renal K^+ excretion in the presence of aldosterone deficiency. Hyperkalemia alters the reabsorption of NH_4^+ in substitution for K^+ in the $Na^+K^+2Cl^-$ cotransporter (NKCC2) in the thick ascending Henle's loop. Hypoaldosteronism reduces the reabsorption of Na^+ and the excretion of K^+, H^+, and NH_4^+ mechanisms that participate in the development and persistence of metabolic acidosis with hyperkalemia, which characterize type IV renal tubular acidosis [33–36].

The close relationship of acid-base and potassium metabolism becomes relevant during certain pathological scenarios, like during the cation exchange involving Na^+, HCO_3^-, H^+, and K^+ molecules, subjected to exchange from ECF to ICF and vice versa, acting as buffer mechanism in the presence of systemic acidosis or alkalosis [26].

A similar scheme occurs along the nephron, for example, K^+ molecules occupy the H^+ binding sites in different transporter proteins, either in the apical and basolateral membranes of the cells of the brush border in the proximal tubule, loop of Henle, and in the principal and α-intercalated cells, in cases of increased $[K^+]s$, to increase K^+ renal excretion.

Some transporter proteins involved in this physiological process are NHE, NKCC2, $HCO_3^-/Cl,^-H^+ATPase$, $H^+K^+ATP'ase$, as well as the pacemaker channels HCN1-HCN3, and the glycoproteins Rhesus: Rhbg, Rhgc, etc. [37–40].

Under physiological conditions, the excess of protons from the intermediate metabolism are excreted as a buffer solution containing equal amounts of NH_3/NH_4^+ and titratable acidity.

On the other hand, in the presence of systemic metabolic acidosis, the highest excretion of H^+ is ammonia. Also, urinary acidification is increased by the physiological levels of various mineralocorticoids.

Usually, during sustained hyperkalemia or systemic acidosis, there is an increase in NH_4^+ excretion, whereas chronic hypokalemia or alkalosis stimulates the opposite effect.

Nonetheless, the clinical interpretation of these mechanisms must be individualized in each case. For example, in cases with Type I or II RTA, hypokalemia will always be present. The same happens in cases of chronic systemic acidosis who have extrarenal potassium losses, as occurs in children with severe diarrhea lasting several days. These patients have metabolic acidosis, due to loss of bicarbonate, but they do develop hypokalemia as well, secondary to total body K^+ depletion [41].

In patients with RTA IV, there is a reduction in the excretion of bicarbonate. This may be the reason why the urine pH can be ≤5.5, adding that the distal tubular excretory capacity for $NH_4{}^+$ remains intact.

In view that citrate excretion is high in Type IV RTA and Ca^{2+} reabsorption is reduced, children with this disease are protected from the development of nephrocalcinosis or nephrolithiasis. These factors mentioned before have a protective effect and avoid hypercalciuria and, consequently, crystallization and deposition of calcium oxalate salts [42].

Table 10.1 shows some of the relevant factors participating in renal tubular K^+ excretion in the principal and α-intercalated cells of the cortical and medullary connector and collector tubules.

Clinical Alterations Related to the Production and Renal Tubular Activity of Aldosterone

The development and, in some cases, the persistence of RTA IV are due to the presence of diverse pathogenic mechanisms, linked to the electrolyte imbalance appearing as a reduction in aldosterone production (hypoaldosteronism), or a lack of response of the renal tubules to the action of aldosterone, thus hindering Na^+ reabsorption and K^+ excretion (pseudohypoaldosteronism).

The pathophysiological mechanisms of some frequent clinical entities are reviewed below. This chapter does not consider all possible entities with hyperkalemia, but only those with RTA Type IV, most linked to hypoaldosteronism or pseudohypoaldosteronism. These diseases show hyperchloremic renal tubular acidosis, with a normal anion gap $[Na^+] - ([HCO_3^-] + [Cl^-])$: 12 ± 2; failure to thrive and hyperkalemia.

Table 10.2 shows the etiology of cases of RTA Type IV.

Table 10.2 Etiology of RTA Type IV

Classification
Aldosterone deficiency
Aldosterone deficiency without kidney alterations (primary adrenal insufficiency)
Addison's disease
Bilateral adrenalectomy
Syndrome of congenital adrenal hyperplasia
(21- hydroxylase deficiency)
Isolated hypoaldosteronism
Isolated hypoaldosteronism in critical illnesses
Hereditary deficiency of corticosterone methyl-oxidase

Table 10.2 (continued)

Hyporeninemia (hypoaldosteronism syndrome)
Diabetes
Gout
Pyelonephritis
Tubulointerstitial nephritis
Nephrosclerosis
Decreased response to aldosterone activity
Pseudo-hypoaldosteronism
Childhood pseudo-hypoaldosteronism
Chronic salt-wasting tubulointerstitial nephritis
Obstructive uropathy
Drugs
Spironolactone
Heparin
Amiloride
Eplerenone
Prostaglandin inhibitors
Triamterene
Captopril
Cyclosporine
Decreased response to aldosterone with selective deficiency
Selective tubular dysfunction with hypertension associated with renin dysfunction
Chronic tubulointerstitial nephritis with chronic kidney disease
Obstructive uropathy
Renal transplantation
Systemic lupus erythematosus
Acute glomerulonephritis
Renal amyloidosis
Non-classified type IV RTA
Distal tubular dysfunction
Renal amyloidosis
Lupus nephritis with anti-basement membrane antibodies
Renal vein thrombosis
Antibiotics: Methicillin, etc.
Factors that contribute or aggravate RTA type IV
KCl supplements
Heparin
Potassium-sparing diuretics
Prostaglandin inhibitors
Captopril
Cyclosporine

Primary hypoaldosteronism, with a normal glomerular filtration rate, results from a deficiency in aldosterone production, often due to surgical ablactation or diseases of the adrenal glands, ending in lack of production of the hormone.

The increase in $[K^+]$s depends on the degree of aldosterone deficiency, leading to renal sodium losses and potassium retention, in turn, due to a decrease in the production of Na^+K^+ATPase. Acidosis per se increases $[K^+]_{ECF}$, due to the cation exchange between ICF and ECF in a systemic buffering mechanism, as a response to the accumulation of H^+ in the ECF. Hyperkalemia reduces ammonium synthesis and reduces the renal tubular reabsorption of HCO_3^-, a mechanism that contributes to the worsening of acidosis [43, 44].

Primary hypoaldosteronism is a deficiency in aldosterone activity or synthesis, clinically manifesting as RTA Type IV. An etiology in children may be adrenal aplasia or hypoplasia with adrenal insufficiency (Addison's disease). In older children, autoimmune dysplasia, hemorrhage, or infections like (mycosis, tuberculosis, etc.) of the adrenal glands, as well as amyloidosis and lupus erythematosus may lead to adrenal insufficiency [44].

Certain rare inherited disorders, such as the deficiency of the enzyme 21-α-hydroxylase of the cholesterol-mineralocorticoid cascade (inherited as an autosomal recessive pattern) cause congenital adrenal hyperplasia syndrome or adrenogenital syndrome, disorders that could be detected during the neonatal period [45, 46].

The clinical manifestations of this syndrome are heterogenous, but mostly predominate ambiguous genitalia with virilization, frequently with Type IV RTA, hyperkalemia, metabolic acidosis, and renal tubular salt wasting. The latter is accompanied by frequent episodes of dehydration [47].

Congenital adrenal hyperplasia is a group of alterations in the steroid biosynthesis from cholesterol, ending in the manufacture of glucocorticoids, mineralocorticoids, and sex hormones. The most frequent alteration is the deficiency of the enzyme 21 α-hydroxylase, which is located in the CYP21 gene and prevents the conversion of 17-hydroxyprogesterone to 11-deoxycortisol, thus avoiding the production of the adrenocorticotropin- hormone (ACTH). This hormone generates an accumulation of the precursors of cortisol and androgens, ending up in virilization in utero [48].

In addition to the enzyme 21 α-hydroxylase, other enzymes may be altered, with diverse clinical manifestations, such as the enzyme 11-β-hydroxylase or the 3-β-hydroxysteroid dehydrogenase [44, 49].

Besides metabolic acidosis, hyperkalemia, and ambiguous genitalia, seen with the deficiency of the enzyme 21 α-hydroxylase, frequent periods of dehydration and hyponatremia may occur. Whereas, in the deficiency of the 11-β-hydroxylase enzyme, there is an accumulation of deoxycorticosterone (DOC). This hormone leads to renal tubular salt retention and secondary arterial hypertension.

Patients with mild chronic renal failure may develop Type IV RTA, frequently showing hyperreninemic hypoaldosteronism syndrome, with hyperchloremic metabolic acidosis, reduced plasma aldosterone concentration, and low renin plasma activity, mild reduction of the GFR (not consistent with the degree of hyperkalemia), and without depletion of the circulating volume [50].

Hyperreninemic hypoaldosteronism syndrome is common in patients with diabetes mellitus, kidney diseases associated with tubulointerstitial nephritis, mild chronic renal failure, obstructive uropathy, post-renal transplantation, amyloidosis, and monoclonal gammopathies, among others [51, 52].

Some conditions, such as diabetes mellitus, chronic kidney failure, obstructive uropathy, lupus erythematosus, and other conditions involving tubulointerstitial nephritis, occasionally have a lack of tubular renal response to physiological or elevated levels of aldosterone (acquired pseudo-hypoaldosteronism), accompanied by renal salt loss, moderate hyperchloremic metabolic acidosis, hyperkalemia, hyponatremia, and recurrent episodes of dehydration. Patients taking K^+-sparing diuretics, such as spironolactone, triamterene, amiloride, eplerenone, and medications such as heparin, prostaglandin inhibitors, captopril, and, cyclosporine, may show the same symptoms [53].

In cases of pseudohypoaldosteronism, the adrenal glands synthesize and secrete aldosterone normally, but the kidneys are not able to respond, due to dissimilar etiologies.

There is recent information about cases with pseudohypoaldosteronism in which new genetic mutations have been described, providing clues about the etiology of these clinical entities, as it happens with Type I pseudo-hypoaldosteronism (PHAI). This disease has two hereditary patterns; one is the autosomal recessive form, with mutations of the epithelial sodium channels, ENaC (SCNN1A, SCNN1B, SCNN1G).

However, most cases are attributed to the mineralocorticoid receptor (MR) mutations, with an autosomal dominant inheritance pattern (NR3C2).

The autosomal recessive phenotype has a more severe clinical presentation than the autosomal dominant phenotype and does not evolve toward spontaneous improvement in the adolescent stage, as frequently occurs with the autosomal dominant phenotype cases. Patients with the PHAI mutation show metabolic acidosis, hyperkalemia, increased aldosterone concentration, and a lack of renal tubular response to aldosterone, with renal tubular sodium loss [54, 55].

Type II pseudohypoaldosteronism (PHAII) is transmitted as an autosomal dominant pattern; the clinical presentation is arterial hypertension, normal peripheral renin activity, normal or elevated plasma aldosterone levels, hyperkalemia, and metabolic acidosis, with normal glomerular filtration rate [56].

The patients with this entity have no renal tubular response to aldosterone activity, due to mutations genetically transmitted as a dominant pattern, located in the lysine-free genes WNK1 and WNK4, encoded in the chromosomes 12 and 17 respectively, or in the KLHL3 gene, the latter as an autosomal recessive transmission trait. The term has its origin in the English language (WNK: "with no lysine kinases"). The WNK1 (PHIIC) and WNK4 (PHAIIB) genes regulate the Na^+ Cl^- cotransporter proteins (NCC), as well as the potassium channel (ROMK), the latter with the capability to exchange K^+ for hydrogen (NH_4^+), in the distal renal tubule.

These genetic mutations cause an increase in Na^+Cl^- (NCC) reabsorption in the NDSA. By reducing the degree of electronegativity in the lumen of the collecting tubule, various physiological mechanisms are triggered, such as the secretion of potassium and retention of protons (NH_4^+) are reduced; the distal chloride flow is increased (Cl^--short-circuit), a Type IV RTA develops with sodium-dependent arterial hypertension, hyperkalemia, mild hyperchloremic metabolic acidosis, with reduced plasma renin activity and reduced aldosterone concentration.

Some patients who develop hypercalciuria may have dental alterations, in addition to mental retardation, muscle weakness, and sodium retention with circulatory volume expansion, and secondarily, arterial hypertension, usually severe.Patients with WNK mutations respond rapidly to the administration of thiazide diuretics. Synonyms to the WNK mutations are high blood pressure with familial hyperkalemia or Gordon disease, and chloride short circuit syndrome (chloride shunt) [57–60].

Differential Diagnosis of Hypoaldosteronism and Pseudo-Hypoaldosteronism

Frame with an algorithm is shown below to describe clinical and laboratory signs and symptoms useful for the differential diagnosis.

Different laboratory techniques may help to diagnose the etiology of the hyperchloremic metabolic acidosis with normal anion gap and hyperkalemia, such as fractional excretion of the filtered potassium (FEK^+), urine Na^+/K^+ ratio; aldosterone concentration in blood and urine, etc. However, the interpretation of the results is difficult, which limits the use of these techniques (Fig. 10.2). Measurement of $[K^+]$ in blood and urine is not useful in the differential diagnosis of hyperkalemia, since the electrolyte concentrations in the urine vary with the amount of H_2O, increasing or reducing the urinary osmolality.

A technique in current use is the determination of the renal transtubular potassium gradient, according to the following formula:

$$\mathrm{GTTK} = \left[\mathrm{K}^+\right]\mathrm{u} / \left[\mathrm{K}^+\right]\mathrm{s} \times \mathrm{Osm_s} / \mathrm{Osm_u}$$

where:

GTTK = renal trans-tubular potassium gradient.

$[K^+]u$: urinary potassium concentration.

$[K^+]_s$: concentration of potassium in the blood.

Osm_s: blood osmolality.

Osm_u: urinary osmolality.

There has been a discrepancy in the results on the GTTK values performed in the clinical case series in patients with hypokalemia and hyperkalemia.

Generally speaking, it is considered that a GTTK value <2 in patients with hypokalemia indicates that there are renal losses of K^+. On the other hand, in cases with hyperkalemia, a GTTK >8 indicates normal bioactivity of aldosterone, and the

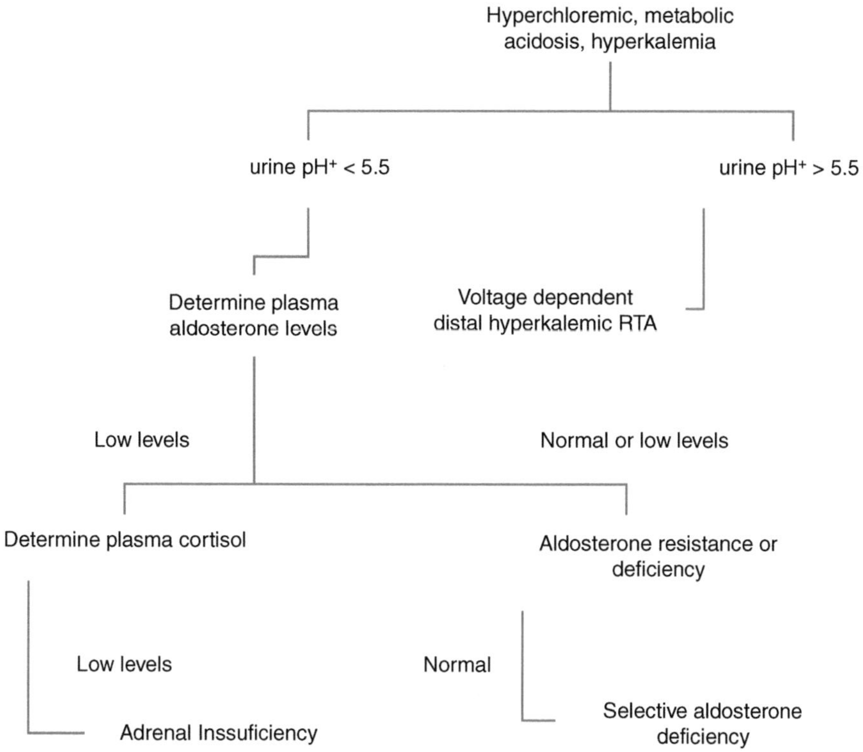

Fig. 10.2 Alghortim for the differential diagnosis of hypoaldosteronism and pseudo-hypoaldosteronism

collecting tubule is having an adequate response to mineralocorticoids. On the other hand, a value of GTTK <6, in the presence of hyperkalemia, indicates a deficiency or resistance to aldosterone.

Since the distal Na^+ load is an important factor in renal K^+ excretion, the $[Na^+]_u$ must be >10 mmol/l, and the urine osmolality must be higher than the blood osmolality: $(Osm_u) \geq (Osm_s)$, because the presence of the antidiuretic hormone (ADH) is important for the secretion of K^+ in the collecting tubule [61–63].

Furthermore, the measurement of GTTK in patients with hyperkalemia facilitates the differential diagnosis between aldosterone deficiency and renal resistance to its activity when an increase in GTTK is observed after the administration of mineralocorticoids. A physiological dose of mineralocorticoids in patients with adrenal insufficiency showed an increase in GTTK >6, about 2 to 6 hours after the administration [64].

At pediatric age, GTTK values <4.1 in children and >4.9 in preschool children indicate reduced aldosterone bioactivity. These values were found at the third percentile in a clinical study that included 473 children with a normal $[K^+]$ for age. Thirteen children with a diagnosis of hypoaldosteronism or pseudo-hypoaldosteronism had GTTK values between 1.6 and 4.1 [65].

In summary, the GTTK result of 6 in adults with hyperkalemia indicates low renal potassium excretion, which corresponds to a GTTK of 4 in older children and 5 in preschoolers [64, 65].

Management and Treatment of ATR IV

Treatment begins with attention to hyperkalemia according to its severity and with the information obtained from the clinical history and the laboratory results.

The reduction of $[K^+]_s$ is based on the use of loop diuretics, such as furosemide and bumetanide; inhaled β-adrenergic agonists (salbutamol), intravenous polarizing solutions, calcium gluconate (cardio-protective), sodium bicarbonate, and cation exchange resins. Furosemide, in addition to inhibiting tubular reabsorption of K^+, facilitates the correction of acidosis by increasing the sodium distal load to the distal convoluted and collector tubules, and consequently, increases the excretion of NH_4^+.

In severe cases, the use of fludrocortisone is recommended, which activates the mineralocorticoid receptors (MR) and increases the activity of the ENaC channels in the connecting and collecting tubules, improving epithelial Na^+ reabsorption, as well as the K^+ and H^+ secretion [66, 67].

In cases with hypoaldosteronism secondary to adrenal insufficiency, treatment consists of the supplementary administration of mineralocorticoids, which correct electrolytic disorders and acid-base metabolism.

In cases of pseudo-hypoaldosteronism, the administration of sodium chloride is sufficient; however, the administration of sodium bicarbonate is required in some cases [68]. Patients with PHA II secondary to WNK mutations respond to thiazide administration [69].

It is recommended to be cautious when treating a diabetic patient with polarizing solutions due to the risk of hyperglycemia and keep a balance of blood glucose levels and insulin administration. Caution is also advised with the administration of sodium bicarbonate, due to the potential development of hypervolemia and hypernatremia [70].

Also, the potassium intake in the diet must be reduced. Early furosemide administration is frequently required to enhance potassium excretion. Also, treatment with fludrocortisone may be considered to increase renal potassium excretion, thus reducing total body potassium [71, 72]. Fludrocortisone simulates the activity of aldosterone by increasing the activity of the ENaC (sodium channels) in the luminal membrane and Na^+K^+ATPase in the basolateral membrane of the principal cells, therefore increasing the reabsorption of Na^+ in exchange for H^+ secretion. This effect is enhanced since fludrocortisone activates H^+ATP'ase, which favors the secretion of hydrogen as NH_4^+ and titratable acidity [31, 73].

Prognosis

The prognosis depends on the etiology, the severity of the case, adherence to treatment, and other factors.

Pseudo-hypoaldosteronism is limited to the age of 4–5 years, subsiding spontaneously. Primary adrenal injuries require permanent supplementation.

The toxicity caused by medications disappears after drug withdrawal.

Hyporeninemic hypoaldosteronism caused by tubulointerstitial nephritis may occur in adult patients with diabetes mellitus and hyperuricemia, so the prognosis is associated with the severity of chronic kidney disease [73].

References

1. Chan JCM, Mak RHK. Acid-base homeostasis. En: Avner ED, Harmon WE, Niaudet P. eds., Pediatric nephrology, 5th ed., Lippincott Williams & Wilkins, Philadelphia, 2004:189–208.
2. Halperin ML, Kamel KS, Goldstein MB. Polyuria. In: Halperin ML, Kamel KS, Goldstein MB, editors. Fluid, electrolyte, and acid-base physiology. 4th ed. Philadelphia: Saunders Elsevier; 2010. p. 403–22.
3. Jorgensen PL. Structure, function and, regulation of Na+, K+-ATPase in the kidney. Kidney Int. 1986;29:10–20.
4. Nakhoul NL, Hamm LL. Vacuolar H+ATPase in the kidney. J Nephrol. 2002;15(Suppl 5):S22–31.
5. Velazquez H, Perazella MA, Wright FS, Ellison DH. Renal mechanism of trimethoprim induced hyperkalemia. Ann Intern Med. 1993;119:296–301.
6. Kleyman TR, Roberts C, Ling BN. A mechanism for pentamidine-induced hyperkalemia: inhibition of distal nephron sodium transport. Ann Intern Med. 1995;122:103–6.
7. Hanukoglu I, Hanukoglu A. Epithelial sodium channel (ENaC) family: phylogeny, structure-function, tissue distribution, and associated inherited diseases. Gene. 2016;579(2):95–132. https://doi.org/10.1016/j.gene.2015.12.061. PMC 4756657. PMID 26772908.
8. Silver RB, Mennit PA, Satlin LM. Stimulation of H^+, K^+ ATPase in intercalated cells of cortical collecting duct with chronic metabolic acidosis. Am J Phys. 1996;270:F539–47.
9. Gamba G. Molecular physiology and pathophysiology of electroneutral cation-chloride cotransporters. Physiol Rev. 2005;85(2):423–93. https://doi.org/10.1152/physrev.00011.2004
10. Aker S, Heering P, Kinne-Saffran E, Deppe C, Grabensee B, Kinne RK. Different effects of cyclosporine a and FK506 on potassium transport systems in MDCK cells. Exp Nephrol. 2001;9:332–40.
11. Kohda Y, Ding W, Phan E, Housini I, Wang J, Star RA, Huang CL. Localization of the ROMK potassium channel to the apical membrane of distal nephron in rat kidney. Kidney Int. 1998;54:1214–23.
12. Melo Z, Cruz-Rangel S, Bautista R, Vázquez N, Castañeda-Bueno M, Mount DB, Gamba G. Molecular evidence for a role for K + -Cl − cotransporters in the kidney. Am J Physiol Renal Physiol. 2013;305(10):F1402–11. https://doi.org/10.1152/ajprenal.00390.2013
13. Grimm PR, Sansom SC. BK channels in the kidney. Curr Opin Nephrol Hypertens. 2007;16(5):430–6.

14. Kamel KS, Ethier JH, Richardson RM, Bear RA, Halperin ML. Urine electrolytes and osmolality: when and how to use them. Am J Nephrol. 1990;10:89–102.
15. Jo D. Renin-angiotensin system in the control of aldosterone secretion. In: Fisher JW, editor. Kidney hormones. New York: Academic Press; 1971. p. 173–205; 3. Mulroy PJ. The adrenal cortex. In Comroe Jr. JH, Alto P, editors. Annual review of physiology. Annual Reviews Inc.; 1972. p. 409–24.
16. Vallés PG, Batlle D. Hypokalemic distal renal tubular acidosis. Adv Chronic Kidney Dis. 2018;25(4):303–20.
17. Halperin ML, Kamel KS. Potassium. Lancet. 1998;352:135–42.
18. Spat A, Hunyady L. Control of aldosterone secretion: a model for convergence in cellular signaling pathways. Physiol Rev. 2004;84:489–539.
19. Palmer LG, Antonian L, Frindt G. Regulation of the Na-K pump of the rat cortical collecting tubule by aldosterone. J Gen Physiol. 1993;102:43–57.
20. Chen SY, Bhargava A, Mastroberardino L, et al. Epithelial sodium channel regulated by aldosterone-induced protein SGK. Proc Natl Acad Sci U S A. 1999;96:2514–9.
21. Vallon V, Wulff P, Huang DY, et al. Role of SGK1 in salt and potassium homeostasis. Am J Physiol Regul Integr Comp Physiol. 2005;288:R4–R10.
22. Lang F, Stournaras C, Alesutan I. Regulation of transport across cell membranes by the serum- and glucocorticoid-inducible kinase SGK1. Mol Membr Biol. 2014;31:29–36.
23. Loffing J, Flores SY, Staub O. Sgk kinases and their role in epithelial transport. Annu Rev Physiol. 2006;68:461–90.
24. Pearce LR, Sommer EM, Sakamoto K, Wullschleger S, Alessi DR. Protor-1 is required for efficient mTORC2-mediated activation of SGK1 in the kidney. Biochem J. 2011;436:169–79.
25. Minuth WW, Gross P, Gilbert P, Kashgaria M. Expression of the a-subunit of Na/K-ATPase in renal collecting duct epithelium during development. Kidney Int. 1987;31:1104–12.
26. Tannen RL. Potassium disorders. In: Kokko JP, Tannen RL, editors. Fluids and electrolytes. Philadelphia: WB Saunders; 1986. p. 150.
27. Greenbaum LA. Pathophysiology of body fluids and fluid therapy. Electrolyte and acid-base disorders. In: Behrman RE, Kliegman RM, Jenson HB, editors. Nelson textbook of pediatrics. 17th ed. Philadelphia: Saunders; 2004. p. 191–242.
28. Custer JW. Blood chemistries and body fluids. In: Custer JW, Rau RE, editors. Harriet Lane handbook. 18th ed. Philadelphia: Mosby; 2009. p. 677–88.
29. Satlin LM, Schwartz GJ. Metabolism of potassium. En Ichikawa I ed., Pediatric textbook of fluids and electrolytes. Williams & Wilkins, Baltimore; 1990: 89–98.
30. Jones DP, Chesney RW. Tubular function. In: Avner ED, Harmon WE, Niaudet P, editors. Pediatric nephrology. 5th ed. Philadelphia: Lippincott Williams & Wilkins; 2004. p. 45–72.
31. Karet EF. Mechanisms in hyperkalemic renal tubular acidosis. J Am Soc Nephrol. 2009;20:251–4. https://doi.org/10.1681/ASN.2008020166.
32. Bidani A, Tuazon DM, Heming TA. Acid-base disorders. Regulation of whole-body acid-base balance. In: DuBose TD, Hamm LL, editors. Acid-Base and electrolyte disorders. Philadelphia: Saunders; 2002. p. 1–21.
33. Wang B, Wen D, Li H, Wang-France J, Sansom SC. Net K+ secretion in the thick ascending limb of mice on a low-Na, high-K diet. Kidney Int. 2017;92(4):864–75. https://doi.org/10.1016/j.kint.2017.04.009
34. Arruda JA, Batlle DC, Sehy JT, Roseman MK, Baronowski RL, Kurtzman NA. Hyperkalemia and renal insufficiency: role of selective aldosterone deficiency and tubular unresponsiveness to aldosterone. Am J Nephrol. 1981;1(3–4):160–7.
35. Schambelan M, Sebastian A. Type IV renal tubular acidosis: pathogenetic role of aldosterone deficiency and hyperkalemia. Nephrologie. 1985;6(3):135–7.
36. Jones DP, Chesney RW. Tubular function. In: Avner ED, Harmon WE, Niaudet P, editors. Pediatric nephrology. 5th ed. Lippincott Williams & Wilkins, Philadelphia; 2004. p. 45–72.
37. Carrisoza-Gaytan R, Rangel C, Salvador C, Saldaña-Meyer R, Escalona C, Satlin LM, Liu W, Zavilowitz B, Joyce Trujillo J, Bobadilla NA, Escobar LI. The hyperpolarization-activated

cyclic nucleotide-gated HCN2 channel transports ammonium in the distal nephron. Kidney Int. 2011;80:832–40. https://doi.org/10.1038/ki.2011.230.
38. Endeward V, Cartron JP, Ripoche P, Gros G. RhAG protein of the rhesus complex is a CO2 channel in the human red cell membrane. FASEB J. 2008;22:64–73.
39. Weiner ID, Hamm LL. Molecular mechanisms of renal ammonia transport. Annu Rev Physiol. 69: 317–340; Chan JCM, Mak RHK. Acid-base homeostasis. In: Avner ED, Harmon WE, Niaudet P, editors. Pediatric nephrology. 5th ed. Philadelphia: Lippincott Williams & Wilkins; 2004. p. 189–208.
40. Finkel KW, DuBose TD. Metabolic acidosis. In: DuBose TD, Hamm LL, editors. Acid-base and electrolyte disorders. Philadelphia: Saunders; 2002. p. 55–66.
41. McSherry E. Current issues in hydrogen transport. En: Gruskin AB, Norman ME, eds, Pediatric nephrology. Hisham MA. Martinus Nijhoff, 1981: 403–415.
42. Kurtzman NA, White MG, Rogers PW. The effect of potassium and extracellular volume on renal bicarbonate reabsorption. Metabolism. 1973:22–481.
43. Schambelan M, Sebastian A, Biglieri E. Prevalence, pathogenesis, and functional significance of aldosterone deficiency in hyperkalemic patients with chronic renal insufficiency. Kidney Int. 1980:17–89.
44. Berend K. Review of the diagnostic evaluation of Normal anion gap metabolic acidosis. Kid Dis. 2017;3:149–59.
45. Speiser PW, Azziz R, Baskin LS, Ghizzoni L, Hensle TW, Merke DP. Congenital adrenal hyperplasia due to steroid 21-hydroxylase deficiency, En: Endocrine Society clinical practice guideline. J Clin Endocrinol Metab. 2010;95(9):4133–60.
46. Janzen N, Riepe FG, Peter M, Sander S, Steuerwald U, Korsch E, et al. Neonatal screening: identification of children with 11ß-hydroxylase deficiency by second-tier testing. Horm Res Paediatr. 2012;77(3):195–9.
47. Chan LF, Campbell DC, Novoselova TV, Clark AJ, Metherell LA. Whole-exome sequencing in the differential diagnosis of primary adrenal insufficiency in children. Front Endocrinol (Lausanne). 2015;6:113.
48. Gill JR, Santos F, Chan JCM. Disorders of potassium metabolism. En: Kidney electrolyte disorders, Chan JCM, Gill JR. Churchill Livingston, New York, 1990: 137–170.
49. Sánchez MC, Hoffman V, Prieto GS, Hernández RJ, Espinosa G. Renal tubular acidosis type IV as a complication of lupus nephritis. Lupus. 2015;25:307–9.
50. Batlle DC, Arruda JA, Kurtzman NA. Hyperkalemic distal renal tubular acidosis associated with obstructive uropathy. N Engl J Med. 1981;304(7):373–80.
51. Menegussi J, Tatagiba LS, Vianna JGP, Seguro AC, Luchi WM. A physiology-based approach to a patient with kyperkalemic renal tubular acidosis. J Bras Nefrol. 2018;40(4):410–7.
52. DeFronzo RA. Hyperkalemia and hyporeninemic hypoaldosteronism. Kidney Int. 1980;17(1):118.
53. Chang SS, Grunder S, Hanukoglu A, Rosler A, Mathew PM, Hanukoglu I, Schild L, Lu Y, Shimkets RA, Nelson-Williams C, Rossier BC, Lifton RP. Mutations in subunits of the epithelial sodium channel cause salt wasting with hyperkalaemic acidosis, pseudohypoaldosteronism type 1. Nat Genet. 1996;12:248–53.
54. Pujo L, Fagart J, Gary F, Papadimitriou DT, Claes A, Jeunemaitre X, Zennaro MC. Mineralocorticoid receptor mutations are the principal cause of renal type 1 pseudohypoaldosteronism. Hum Mutat. 2007;28:33–40.
55. Geller DS, Zhang J, Zennaro MC, Vallo-Boado A, Rodriguez-Soriano J, et al. Autosomal dominant pseudohypoaldosteronism type 1: mechanisms, evidence for neonatal lethality, and phenotypic expression in adults. J Am Soc Nephrol. 2006;17:1429–36.
56. Julie R. Ingelfinger. Etiology of childhood hypertension. En: Comprehensive pediatric nephrology, 2008 https://doi.org/10.1016/B978-0-323-04883-5.50049-0.
57. Both T, Zietse R, Hoorn EJ, Van Hagen PM, Dalm VASH, Van Laar JAM, Van Daele PLA. Everything you need to know about distal renal tubular acidosis in autoimmune disease. Rheumatol Int. 2014;34:1037–45.

58. New MI, Geller DS, Fallo F, Wilson RC. Monogenic low renin hypertension. Trends Endocrinol Metab. 2005;16(3):92–7.
59. Kahle KT, Wilson FH, Leng Q, Lalioti MD, O'Connell AD, Dong K, Rapson AK, Giebisch G, Hebert SC, Lifton RP. WNK4 regulates the balance between renal NaCl reabsorption and K+ secretion. Nat Genet. 2003;35(4):372–6.
60. Avila Poletti D, De Azevedo L, Iommi C, Heldal K, Musso CG. Hyperchloremic metabolic acidosis in the kidney transplant patient. Postgrad Med. 2019;131(3):171–5.
61. Weinstein AM. A mathematical model of rat cortical collecting duct: determinants of the transtubular potassium gradient. Am J Physiol Renal Physiol. 2001;280:F1072–92.
62. West ML, Marsden PA, Richardson RM, Zettle RM, Halperin ML. New clinical approach to evaluate disorders of potassium excretion. Miner Electrolyte Metab. 1986;12:234–8.
63. Field MJ, Stanton BA, Giebisch GH. Influence of ADH on renal potassium handling: a micropuncture and microperfusion study. Kidney Int. 1984;25:502–11.
64. Choi MJ, Ziyadeh FN. The utility of the Transtubular potassium gradient in the evaluation of hyperkalemia. J Am Soc Nephrol. 2008;19(3):424–6. https://doi.org/10.1681/ASN.2007091017.
65. Rodriguez-Soriano J, Ubetagoyena M, Vallo A. Transtubular potassium concentration gradient: a useful test to estimate renal aldosterone bio-activity in infants and children. Pediatr Nephrol. 1990;4:105–10.
66. Lee J, Moffet BS. Treatment of pediatric hyperkalemia with sodium polystyrene sulfonate. Pediatr Nephrol. 2016;31:2113–7.
67. Villegas-Anzo F, Castellanos-Olivares A, Gracida-Juárez C, Rangel-Montes MA, Espinoza-Pérez R, Cancino-López J. Manejo de la hiperkalemia transoperatoria en pacientes con insuficiencia renal crónica sometidos a trasplante renal. Rev Mex Trans. 2013;2(2):50–7.
68. Santos F, Gil PH, Alvárez AS. Renal tubular acidosis. CurrOpinPediatr. 2017;29(2):206–10.
69. Voyer LA, Caupolican A. Hiperkalemia, Diagnóstico y tratamiento. Arch Argent Pediatr. 2000; 98(5): 337–44.
70. Ruiz-Mejía R, Ortega-Olivares LM, Naranjo-Carmona CA, Suárez-Otero R. Tratamiento de la hipercalemia en pacientes con enfermedad renal crónica en terapia dialítica. Med Int Méx. 2017;33(6):778–96.
71. Kamel KS, Wei C. Controversial issues in the treatment of hyperkalaemia. Nephrol Dial Transplant. 2003;18:2215–8.
72. Dhayat N, Gradwell M, Anderegg M, Schneider L, Luethi D, Mattmann C, et al. Furosemide/fludrocortisone test and clinical parameters to diagnose incomplete distal renal tubular acidosis in kidney stone formers. Clin J Am Soc Nephrol. 2017;12:1507–17.
73. DeFronso RA. Hyperkalemia and hyporeninemic hypoaldosteronism. Nephrology forum. Kidney Int. 1980;7:118–34.

Chapter 11
Renal Tubular Acidosis Due to Miscellaneous Etiology

Mario Matos-Martínez and Ricardo Muñoz

Introduction

Primary or hereditary renal tubular acidosis (RTA) is a syndrome with a heterogeneous etiology and clinical presentation, mainly characterized by hyperchloremic metabolic acidosis with a normal anion gap, and hypokalemia or hyperkalemia. In some cases, nephrocalcinosis, failure to thrive, and occasionally, deafness are observed. This is due to a renal tubular inability to maintain normal HCO_3^- concentration, either due to an inability to reclaim or recover the filtered bicarbonate in the proximal tubule or to an impediment to generating new bicarbonate through net acid renal excretion (NARE) at the distal collecting tubule. In both situations, there is an inadequate renal capacity to acidify the urine to a pH of 6.5.

Recently, some chromosome mutations have been detected in the genes that regulate transporter, cotransporter, and exchange proteins, as well as of the enzymes

M. Matos-Martínez (Deceased)
Pediatric Nephrology Service, Medical Unit of High Specialty National Medical Center La Raza, Mexican Institute of Social Security, Mexico City, Mexico

Faculty of Medicine, National Autonomous University of Mexico, Mexico City, Mexico

R. Muñoz (✉)
Retired from: Department of Pediatric Nephrology, Hemodialysis Unit, The Children's Hospital at Albany Medical Center, Albany, NY, USA

Retired from: Pediatric Nephrology Department, Hospital Infantil de México Federico Gómez, Mexico City, Mexico

Retired from: Research Division, Hospital Infantil de Mexico Federico Gomez, Mexico City, Mexico

Retired from: National System of Investigators, Level I, Mexico City, Mexico

Retired from: North American Pediatric Renal Transplantation Collaborative Study (NAPRTCS) Study, Woburn, MA, USA

R. Muñoz (ed.), *Renal Tubular Acidosis in Children*,
https://doi.org/10.1007/978-3-030-91940-5_11

that catalyze biochemical reactions to form bicarbonate, mainly carbonic anhydrase type II (CA II), although various carbonic anhydrases participate in this process [1–3].

The primary etiology is due to genetic mutations of the transmembrane mechanisms for the transportation of different electrolyte molecules involved in different types of RTA, described in detail in Chap. 4 and other corresponding chapters of this publication.

Some children develop RTA secondary to systemic diseases of diverse etiology, such as some immune entities (Sjögren's syndrome, lupus nephropathy, etc.), that are mentioned in the corresponding chapters; or secondary to the use of drugs; renal immaturity of the preterm newborn; chronic malnutrition, and hereditary diseases (Fanconi's syndrome).

Correction or clinical improvement of the alteration is achieved in some cases, once the offending agent is removed. In this chapter, the mechanisms of some of these etiologies will be reviewed.

It is relevant to mention that these cases present with the typical symptoms and laboratory results of primary RTA. However, the clinical manifestations disappear when the causal factor is removed, which is why they have been called "transient" RTA. In our consideration, however, these patients can not strictly be diagnosed as having true RTA, since they keep intact the mechanisms for urinary acidification.

RTA Secondary to Nephrotoxic Drugs Acting in the Distal Tubule (DRTA)

As mentioned above, some medications may interfere with the normal mechanisms aimed to maintain the normal concentration of HCO_3^- in the body fluids, either by the proximal recovery of bicarbonate or by the distal secretion of hydrogen.

RTA induced by drugs or chemicals has been described since the end of the last century. These substances can affect the carrier proteins that transport, co-transport, or exchange protons and other molecules through the renal tubular cells. This variety of RTA may appear at any age, although children who happen to be more susceptible to some drug's nephrotoxicity are more prone to develop RTA.

The first described clinical observations were in cases that had been treated with certain drugs, such as amphotericin B, vitamin D, lithium salts, methicillin, foscarnet, and amiloride. The later drug works indirectly, by imitating a urinary tract obstruction or by altering the voltage-dependent mechanisms of urinary acidification [4, 5].

The mechanism by which these drugs develop distal RTA may be explained by alterations in the secretion of hydrogen (H^+) ions, or by altering the activity of the Na^+/H^+ and H^+ATPase transport molecules [6]. A distal RTA (Type I) develops due to the nephrotoxicity site of the mentioned drugs,

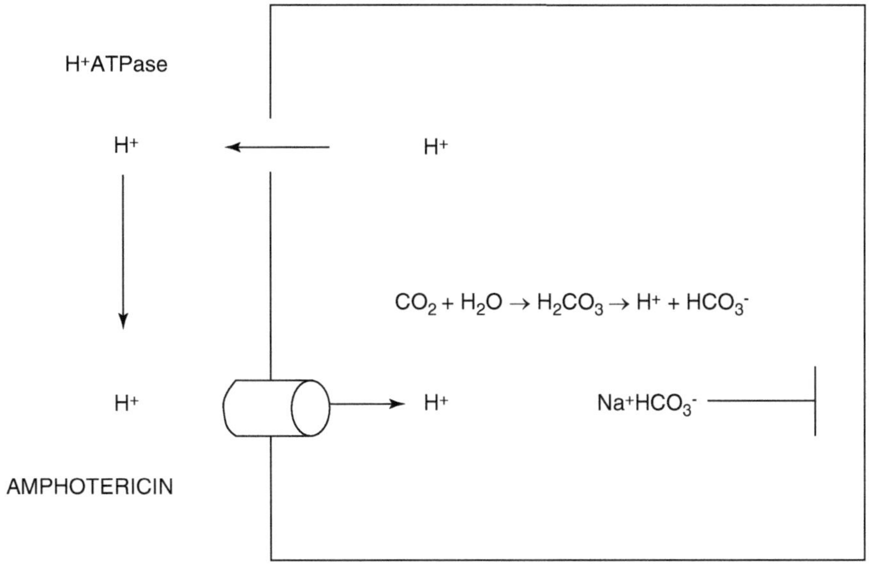

Fig. 11.1 Nephrotoxicity mechanism of amphotericin B in the α-intercalated cells of the collecting and connecting tubules. Amphotericin nephrotoxicity may be the cause of porosity formation in the cell membrane, leading to a back-flow of H^+ ions in a retrograde transfer from the tubular lumen to the cytoplasm. This phenomenon inhibits the excretion of H^+ and reabsorption of HCO_3^- ("new bicarbonate"), leading to the development of RTA

Amphotericin B nephrotoxicity comes up at the α-intercalated cells of the collecting tubules, where it produces porosities in the cell membranes and, a back-flow of hydrogen (H^+) ions into the cytosol, thereby inhibiting H^+ secretion [7]. See Fig. 11.1.

Lithium salts are commonly used to treat some psychiatric disorders, such as compulsive depressive bipolar disease. The mechanism that alters the tubular function to secrete H^+ ions correlates with the development of tubulointerstitial nephritis and hypercalcemia [8].

RTA Secondary to Nephrotoxic Drugs Acting in the Proximal Tubule (PRTA)

The use of nephrotoxic drugs is a frequent cause of Type II RTA, due to the great number of commonly used medications that can inhibit the renal tubular mechanisms in charge of recovering the filtered HCO_3^-, like antibiotics, some diuretics, chemotherapy, and other oncology treatments, immunologic diseases, as well as for the control of epilepsy.

Acetazolamide and other inhibitors of carbonic anhydrase may be a frequent cause of RTA. Type IV carbonic anhydrase (luminal) is necessary for proximal tubular reabsorption of bicarbonate, by promoting the conversion of H_2CO_3 (carbonic acid) into H_2O and CO_3 (equilibrium reaction), and consequently, be reabsorbed into the cytoplasm. The equilibrium reaction will be reversed in the cytosol of the proximal tubular cell (in the presence of carbonic anhydrase Type II (intracellular CA II)), to complete the reabsorption of the filtered bicarbonate in the basolateral membrane. Acetazolamide is used as a diuretic in the treatment of glaucoma, hydrocephalus, and other pathologies, and frequently causes RTA.

Another drug that produces PRTA by inhibiting AC IV is topiramate, which is used in the management of seizures, as well as prophylactic therapy for migraine [9].

Ifosfamide and cyclophosphamide commonly used in patients with malignancies are alkylating agents of the oxazaphosphorines type that can induce nephrotoxicity, mostly in children. In addition to PRTA, these patients may develop a full Fanconi''s syndrome, with glycosuria, aminoaciduria, hyperphosphaturia, hypercalciuria, citraturia, and bicarbonate urine losses, thus, preventing recovery of the filtered HCO_3^-.

Ifosfamide exerts its nephrotoxicity through its metabolites, as it is oxidized by cytochrome P3A5 (CYP3A5) and cytochrome P 2B6 (CYP2B6), which are abundant in kidney tissues. The resulting metabolite is chloride-acetaldehyde(CAA) which causes a dysfunction of the mitochondrial oxidation and phosphorylation in the proximal tubular cell, inhibiting the production of cellular energy and other alterations of the cellular function through complex I (NADH: ubiquinone oxidoreductase) of the mitochondrial respiratory chain [10].

Platinum salts, such as cisplatin, oxaliplatin, and carboxylplatin, induce PRTA by a direct toxic effect on amino acid transporters and, similar to aminoglycosides, inhibit cellular ATP production, usually after prolonged use [11].

Other drugs that may induce nephrotoxicity and PRTA are tetracyclines, streptozocin, azacitidine, mercaptopurine, valproic acid, and ranitidine. Aminoglycosides (gentamicin) enter the proximal cell through the megalin and cubulin system, while tetracyclines do so by the organic anion transporter system. Once inside the cytoplasm, they bind and damage the mitochondrial ribosomes, and interfere with the production of ATP necessary for normal cellular functions [9].

RTA Secondary to Nephrotoxic Drugs Acting in the "Distal Aldosterone-sensitive Nephron" (ASDN)

RTA secondary to the use of drugs that inhibit the aldosterone activity in the "aldosterone sensitive zone" (in the connecting and cortical collecting distal nephron) develops RTA Type IV.

Alterations of the "aldosterone sensitive distal nephron" (ASDN) zone affect the function of the mineralocorticoid activity of aldosterone at the principal cells in this area. The clinical presentation of type IV RTA is systemic metabolic acidosis, low $[Cl^-]$ levels, hyperkalemia, normal anion gap, and normal glomerular filtration rate.

Contrary to what happens in other types of RTA (proximal and distal types), which develop hypokalemia, patients with RTA type IV develop hyperkalemia instead.

Type IV RTA may be due to a reduction in aldosterone production in the zona glomerulosa of the adrenal cortex (hypoaldosteronism), or by a defect in aldosterone activity (pseudohypoaldosteronism), caused by the inhibition of the specific distal tubular cell mineralocorticoid receptor (MR). A variety of medications may cause hypoaldosteronism and hyperkalemia through diverse mechanisms.

Nonsteroidal anti-inflammatory drugs (NSAIDs), β-receptor antagonists, cyclosporin A, tacrolimus, and aliskiren inhibit renin secretion of the Polkissen cells of the juxtaglomerular apparatus and, as a consequence, the conversion of angiotensinogen to angiotensin I.

Another mechanism is the inhibition of some of the biochemical steps of the renin-angiotensin-aldosterone system (RAAS). These mechanisms include drugs that inhibit the enzyme convertase, which physiologically converts angiotensin I to angiotensin II, called ACE inhibitors such as captopril, lisinopril, and enalapril, as well as blockers of the angiotensin II type I receptors (AII R blockers), losartan type.

A third mechanism includes medications that alter the aldosterone metabolism, such as ketoconazole and heparin.

The fourth mechanism includes drugs that directly block the action of aldosterone, like spironolactone and eplerenone. Once aldosterone is blocked, H^+ and K^+ secretion becomes averted, causing metabolic acidosis with hyperkalemia.

Other drugs are responsible for the development of type IV RTA without interference with the RAAS, such as trimethoprim with sulfamethoxazole and pentamidine, which interfere with the reabsorption of Na^+, closing the sodium channels, therefore, inhibiting indirectly the secretion of K^+ and H^+ [12].

RTA Type IV in the Full-term Baby and the Premature Newborn

Childhood is an evolutionary transitional period coming from the species that preceded the human being, throughout childhood and adolescence, until the achievement of adult life. The anatomical and physiological changes that take place during this period, mainly during fetal life and the neonatal period, have a high impact on the function of different organs. The comparison (in absolute terms) of the renal physiology of the adult with that of children, is thus, inappropriate, arising a false consideration that the renal function of the child is immature, when in fact, is a normal physiological function.

The renal functional changes occurring during this period are in agreement with the body needs of the individual, according to age (see Chap. 2). As an example, misinterpretation of the laboratory results of children's blood gases based on the normal adult values is one of the main factors leading to a false diagnosis of RTA in children [20].

The systematic study of renal function in full-term newborns and preterm infants began more than 70 years ago. During pregnancy, the placenta regulates the homeostasis of the fetus, including electrolyte and acid-base balance, in the context of the increased acid load, generated by the metabolism of intrauterine fetal constant growth.

The fetal kidney produces most of the amniotic fluid and this, in turn, favors intrauterine lung development and protects the fetus during the increased fetal development [13].

During human embryogenesis, the pronephros appears around the first 3 weeks of gestation and disappears by apoptosis around the fifth week. From then, up to the twelfth week of gestational age, the mesonephros develops and starts to function in a rudimentary way. The mesonephros is a primitive renal system, from which the metanephros or mature kidney develops.

The renal mass grows exponentially from there on and, it may be visualized in the histological studies of the renal tissue toward the eighteenth gestational week. Nephrogenesis accelerates during the second half of pregnancy and becomes completed at about the 37th week of gestational age [13, 14].

The fetal renal plasma flow increases from 20 ml/min to 60 ml/min from weeks 25 to 40 of gestation. The glomerular filtration rate (GFR) increases in parallel with the growing renal mass as fetal age advances.

At the time of clamping the umbilical cord, important transitional hemodynamic changes occur in the organism, during which the placental organic regulation is transferred to the kidneys.

In the premature newborn this process is more complicated. The hemodynamic changes, including renal blood flow, glomerular filtration rate, as well as of most of the other renal tubular functions are performed with greater difficulty and at a slower speed, compared to the full-term baby [15].

During the neonatal period, there is an increase in the organic acid load due to increased protein metabolism, provided by milk feedings. This, together with bone and body mass growth, leads to a significant increase in hydrogen ion production, from amino acid metabolism.

The premature baby takes longer to make the necessary physiological adjustments to buffer and excrete the acid load [17]. The average concentration of blood bicarbonate [HCO_3^-]p is lower in the term newborn than the adult and older children. This is a normal physiological condition that should be considered to avoid a false diagnosis of systemic metabolic acidosis, and RTA in the newborn baby.

The average HCO_3^- concentration in the full-term newborn is 19.5 mmol/l, with a normal range of 14.5 to 24.5 mmol/l [18]. This physiological phenomenon is due to a reduction of the proximal tubular threshold of HCO_3^- which is normally reduced during childhood, mostly in the newborn.

There is no convincing scientific explanation for this phenomenon. Perhaps, among other causes, the threshold of reabsorption of HCO_3^- is reduced since it is coupled to the proximal tubular reabsorption of Na^+. In turn, Na+ reabsorption in this nephron area depends upon the production of Na^+K^+ATPase, known to be markedly reduced throughout childhood, mainly during the newborn period. Therefore, increased natriuresis and bicarbonate excretion is observed [19]. The lower threshold of sodium bicarbonate reabsorption results in a reduction in the $[HCO_3^-]$p, ensuing in a steady state of physiological metabolic acidosis. This normal clinical scenario should not be confused with a false diagnosis of systemic metabolic acidosis and renal tubular acidosis during childhood [20].

The physiological reduction of the bicarbonate reabsorption threshold in the newborn is partially compensated by a normal or increased capacity for distal excretion of H^+. In absolute and quantitative terms, distal H^+ excretion is lower in the newborn than in older children or adults. However, considering the body weight (in kilograms), the newborn's kidneys can excrete 50 to 100% more acids than the adult; a clinical observation determined in full-term and preterm neonates [21]. Acidification tests carried out in premature infants during the first 6 weeks of life showed a gradual increase in maximum H^+ excretion, which occurred simultaneously with an average increase in $[HCO_3^-]$p from12 mEq/l, to 18–19 mEq/l at the end of the study [21].

RTA Secondary to Severe Caloric-Protein Malnutrition

Pioneering studies of kidney function in malnourished patients at different ages showed that net renal acid excretion was reduced; a phenomenon thought to be due to caloric-protein malnutrition and its negative impact on renal physiology [22]. Subsequently, it was observed that malnourished children, as well as adults, maintain blood pH and $[HCO_3^-]$ within normal limits, even when extra-renal fluid and electrolyte losses occur, as happened in babies with gastroenteritis or, after an exogenous acid load.

Diverse explanations, some contradictory, try to explain this phenomenon. It was inferred that the renal excretion of H^+ is actually due to a decrease in acid production secondary to malnutrition. However, malnourished children conserve their urinary acidification capacity [23, 24].

Another study found that acid excretion in these patients is slightly reduced, possibly secondary to factors that accompany their poor nutritional status, such as hypokalemia [25, 26]. Furthermore, hypophosphatemia reduces the leakage of HPO_4^{2-} as well as titrable urinary acidity, which disappears after phosphate administration [24]. These findings were corroborated in 8 children with severe caloric-protein malnutrition, in whom a normal, albeit slow, ability to excrete H^+ was found, compared to the control group, after an ammonium chloride ($NH_4^+ + Cl^-$) load [27].

References

1. Hamm LL, Nakhoul N, Herin-Smith S. Acid-Base Homeostasis. Clin J Am Nephrol. 2015;10:2232–42.
2. Karet FE. Disorders of water and acid-base homeostasis. Nephron Physiol. 2011;118:28–34.
3. Berend K, de Vries PJ, A, OB Gans R. Physiological approach to assessment of acid-base disturbance. N Engl J Med. 2014;371:1434–45.

4. Curtis MR, Sebastian, Mc Sherry E. Renal acidosis. Kidney Int. 1972;1:322–40.
5. Kurtzman NA. Acquired distal renal acidosis. Kidney Int. 1983;24:807–19.
6. Gil FZ, Malnic G. Effect of amphotericin on renal acidification in rat. Pflügers Arch. 1989;413:280–6.
7. Zietze R, Zoutendijk R, Hoorn EJ. Fluid, electrolyte and acid-base disorders associated with antibiotic therapy. Nat Rev Nephrol. 2009;5:193–202.
8. Grünfeld JP, Rossier B. Lithium nephrotoxicity revisited. Nat Rev Nephrol. 2009;5:270–6.
9. Liamis G, Milionis HJ, Elisaf M. Pharmacologically-induced metabolic acidosis. Drug Saf. 2010;33:371–391a.
10. Nissim I, Horyn O, Daikhin Y, Nissim II, Luhovyy B, Phillips P, Yudkoff M. Ifosfamide-induced nephrotoxicity: mechanism and prevention. Cancer Res. 2006;66:7824–31.
11. Kitterer D, Schwab M, Alscher D, Braun N, Latus J. Drug-induced acid-base disorders. Pediatr Nephrol. 2015;30:1407–23.
12. Wang AM, Schwartz GJ, Alpert SI. Urinary acidification. In: Polin RA, Abman SH, Rowitch DH, Benitz WE, Fox WW, editors. Fetal and neonatal physiology. Philadelphia: Elsevier; 2017. p. 1066–73.
13. Mc Crory WW. Developmental nephrology. Cambridge: Harvard University Press; 1972. p. 40–6.
14. Wolf AS. Embryology. In: Avner ED, Harmon WE, Niaudet P, editors. Pediatric nephrology. 15th ed. Philadelphia: Lippincott Williams & Wilkins; 2004. p. 3–24.
15. Veille JC, Hanson RA, Tatum K, Kelley K. Quantitative assessment of human fetal renal blood flow. Am J Obstet Gynecol. 1993;169:1399–402.
16. Schwartz GJ, Haycock GB, Chir B, Edelmann CM, Spitzer A. Late metabolic acidosis: a reassessment of the definition. J Pediatr. 1979;95:102–7.
17. Chevalier R. Developmental renal physiology of the low birth weight pre – term newborn. J Urol. 1996;156:714–9.
18. Edelmann CM, Gruskin AB, Acosta MI. Renal bicarbonate reabsorption and hydrogen ion excretion in normal infants. J Clin Ivest. 1967;46:1309–7.
19. Baum M, Gattineni J, Satlin M. Postnatal Renal Development. In: Alpern R, Caplan M, Moe N, Seldin, Giebisch's, editors. The kidney. Boston: Elsevier; 2013. p. 911–31.
20. Muñoz RA, Escobar L, Medeiros M. Acidosis tubular renal en niños: conceptos actuales de diagnóstico y tratamiento. Bol Med Hosp Infant Mex. 2013;70. no.3 México may./jun
21. Sulyok E, Heim T. Assessment of maximal urinary acidification in premature infants. Biol Neonate. 1971;19:200–2010.
22. Klahr S, Alleyne G. Effects of chronic protein-calorie malnutrition on the kidney. Kidney Int. 1973;3:129–41.
23. Alleyne G. The effect of severe protein caloric malnutrition on the renal function of Jamaican children. Pediatrics. 1967;39:400–11.
24. Edelman CM, Houston IB, Soriano JB, Biochis H, Stark H. Renal excretion of hydrogen ion in children with idiopathic growth retardation. J Pediatr. 1968;72:443–51.
25. Smith R. Urinary acidification defect in chronic infantile malnutrition. Lancet. 1959;i:764.
26. Waterlow JC, Wills V. Balance studies in malnourished Jamaican infants. 1 absorption and retention of nitrogen and phosphorus. Br J Nutr. 1960;14:183–98.
27. Paniagua R, Santos D, Muñoz R, Luengas J, Frenk S. Renal function in protein-energy malnutrition. Pediatr Res. 1980;14:1260–2.

Correction to: Physiology of Renal Potassium Handling

Adrián Rafael Murillo-de-Ozores, Gerardo Gamba, and María Castañeda-Bueno

Correction to:
Chapter 3 in: R. Muñoz (eds.), *Renal Tubular Acidosis in Children*, https://doi.org/10.1007/978-3-030-91940-5_3

The affiliation details of the authors in Chapter 3 were incorrectly published. The initially published version has now been corrected.

The correct affiliations are below:

Adrián Rafael Murillo-de-Ozores
Departamento de Nefrología y Metabolismo Mineral
Instituto Nacional de Ciencias Médicas y Nutrición Salvador Zubirán
Mexico City, Mexico

Gerardo Gamba
Departamento de Nefrología y Metabolismo Mineral
Instituto Nacional de Ciencias Médicas y Nutrición Salvador Zubirán
Mexico City, Mexico

María Castañeda Bueno
Departamento de Nefrología y Metabolismo Mineral
Instituto Nacional de Ciencias Médicas y Nutrición Salvador Zubirán
Mexico City, Mexico

The updated original version of this chapter can be found at
https://doi.org/10.1007/978-3-030-91940-5_3

R. Muñoz (ed.), *Renal Tubular Acidosis in Children*,
https://doi.org/10.1007/978-3-030-91940-5_12

Index

R. Muñoz (ed.), *Renal Tubular Acidosis in Children*,
https://doi.org/10.1007/978-3-030-91940-5

GPSR Compliance

The European Union's (EU) General Product Safety Regulation (GPSR) is a set of rules that requires consumer products to be safe and our obligations to ensure this.

If you have any concerns about our products, you can contact us on ProductSafety@springernature.com

In case Publisher is established outside the EU, the EU authorized representative is:

Springer Nature Customer Service Center GmbH
Europaplatz 3
69115 Heidelberg, Germany

Batch number: 10732090

Printed by Printforce, the Netherlands